ANCIENT WISDOM
FOR CHANGING TIMES

ANCIENT WISDOM
FOR CHANGING TIMES

THE MASTER'S GIFT TO THE WORLD

UNITING WITH YOUR INNER WISDOM
THROUGH THE POWER OF THE BREATH
*CHANGE YOUR BREATHING AND CHANGE
YOUR LIFE*

A Guide for Developing, Storing, and Manifesting Your Energy

BY SIFU JIM BEASLEY AND SIFU JEFF LARSON

To order additional copies of this book, contact:
Xlibris Corporation
1-888-795-4274
www.Xlibris.com
Orders@Xlibris.com
121089

CONTENTS

INTRODUCTION

SINCE THE ADVENT of Western medicine, especially as it exists today, medical practice has focused its efforts on the treatment of disease. Huge advances in diagnostics and physiology have allowed health practitioners to provide patients with cutting-edge cures for diseases once thought incurable. Examples of the wonders of modern medicine can be found in the eradication of smallpox as a disease, the fact that cancers have been shrunk with multimodal chemotherapeutics, and the use of chimeric antibodies to pinpoint and target specific bacteria.

The achievements and discoveries of Western Medicine and modern medical research have changed and improved our daily lives. From the advent of aspirin to the discovery of penicillin and targeted pain medications, we see evidence of modern medicine's ability to improve our quality of life, including its ability to sustain and even prolong life itself. What Western medicine has lacked, however, is the holistic approach to disease prevention which health practitioners in the East have known about and used successfully for thousands of years.

Since the Yellow Emperor's classic text on internal medicine, written around 2,600 BC and believed to be the origin of Eastern medicine, Eastern physicians have studied and mapped energy pathways in the body and learned how stagnation and blockages of this energy can lead to illness. This understanding of the natural harmony of energy pathways in the body has led to a holistic and preventative approach to illness which pervades Eastern culture.

Of all the preventative practices discussed within Eastern medicine, Qigong (pronounced "*chee kung*") is considered to be one of the most powerful and beneficial wellness programs. Qigong enhances our natural breathing process by teaching us to inhale and exhale more efficiently. Some Qigong programs further enhance our breathing patterns by adding relaxed, flowing movements which facilitate healthy energy flow throughout the body along the natural pathways or meridians. These simple Qigong exercises help prevent (and even clear) energy blockages and thus promote health and wellness. The movements themselves are often very simple and easy to perform, so they can be practiced by a person of any age or body type.

As a surgeon and practitioner of Qigong, these two seemingly opposite approaches have made a dramatic impact on my health, my perspective, and how I practice medicine. Qigong practice increases vitality, stimulates the healthy flow of blood throughout the body, and promotes health and wellness. In addition, Qigong uses the body's own physiology to slow the effects of aging, as evidenced in the rosy cheeks and healthy glow of long-time Qigong practitioners.

The simple movements work to naturally fight disease by gently cleansing and oxygenating the internal organs

I believe that Qigong can improve hypertension, decrease the effects of atherosclerosis, and increase blood flow, combating peripheral vascular disease. As one practices Qigong, even for a few minutes each day, you find that you have increased energy throughout the day, that you are able to focus better, and that you experience an overall improved sense of health.

Qigong has not only benefited me physically, the benefit I gain from the quiet, contemplative Moments of my daily practice have made me a better surgeon, husband, and father, and has provided me with a relaxing, enjoyable practice which I will be able to do regardless of my age.

Sifu Larson has been an incredible teacher and inspiration. I have always enjoyed his stories, his sense of history, and the deep well of knowledge he possesses regarding Qigong and its many benefits. I cannot recommend his work highly enough and I encourage everyone to try Qigong for themselves and to experience first-hand the sense of greater health and vitality.

Chris Carlson M.D., surgical oncologist

In the West, in spite of our tremendous progress, we are experiencing a medical crisis. Even the most conservative doctors agree that people have become too dependent on their doctors and medications to stay healthy. No matter how competent our government or our medical system becomes, it cannot completely heal us or keep us well.

Gradually we have given away our power to heal ourselves. Ideally, healing should be our job. Doctors and medication can help, but we should be doing our own work, and more of it. It is hard to take back our power to self-heal when we are faced in all directions with the latest breakthrough health program.

Even the experts often directly contradict each other, with regards to diet, for example. There are so many choices that it is hard to know what direction to go in. This also brings us additional stress, and the more we depend on medications to solve the problem, the greater our stress becomes. This burden, however, is significantly lessened when we learn the secrets of how to heal ourselves.

Taking back the responsibility to heal ourselves is the answer to our healthcare crisis.

As we learn to awaken within ourselves our natural self-healing ability, we no longer feel confused about which health program is right for us. We gain confidence in our ability to heal ourselves through finding and working with the right programs.

Doctors continually find that what works for one person does not work for another. It is often a mystery why one program works for many but not all. The answer to this question lies in understanding how the body heals itself, which the body is perfectly designed to do. That is why some people stay healthy.

When we get sick, a part of our natural self-help healing response is blocked or suppressed in some way. If we learn to awaken our chi through Floating Monk Qigong and other alternative healing methods, we have a better chance of helping ourselves return to balance and wellness.

Already, doctors in the West have come to recognize the amazing benefits of six thousand-year-old traditional Chinese medicine. Most have come to recognize and accept the value of Chinese acupuncture.

Great Masters and teachers of all traditions have spoken of a time when the secrets would come forth, a time when humankind would be able to realize the higher truths about the life we have been given so everyone could live in wellness, justice, and harmony. The time is now. The shift has taken place.

In my own way, I have sifted through these many approaches and used what works for me. The result was clearly a blessed life with much love and success, and yes, my blindness was healed. Because of my years of disciplined practice, I was given access to many of the most advanced techniques which I, in turn, kept secret.

About three years ago, I began to notice that people's self-healing results were much more profound than in previous years. I discovered that people progressed more quickly in these different practices when they moved from the beginning techniques and into the advanced techniques.

I discovered that people only need access to the secrets to receive benefits, which until now, only the Masters have enjoyed. In times past, these advanced techniques were kept secret because they did not work for the average person, but that is not true anymore.

Sifu Jeff Larson has spent his life studying and mastering Qigong and Kung Fu. His years of dedicated study have allowed him to become an Enter the Gate Disciple of Grand Master Henry Poo Yee, and a Certified Black Sash in Qigong and Kung Fu. He has been featured in *Inside Kung Fu Magazine*, on the *Nadia Sahari Show*, and as a special guest on the *Health Matters* radio show. He is a self-healing pioneer who has trained hundreds of people in Floating Monk Qigong techniques and who offers insights that were only available in the past to a select few. He gives you access to information and techniques that would otherwise be unattainable. I have personally benefited from many of Sifu Jeff's power-healing secrets. In one session with his assistance, I released chronic low back pain which I had experienced for more than thirty years.

With Sifu Jeff making these programs available to the general public for the first time, you can now learn to use the Floating Monk Qigong techniques to heal yourself. These simple, invigorating programs can be used by young and old, lay and professionals alike.

Experience the benefit of these programs by doing a brief, relaxing daily Qigong practice. I am excited to be involved in sharing this information with others who can and benefit from it. Use these practices to self-heal physical, mental, emotional, and spiritual conditions. Now that Sifu Jeff, with the Master's permission, has made this information available to the public, you too can use these simple and practical self-healing tools to restore your own health.

Stay bright in the light,

Sifu Mark Armstrong, OMD

(The Pace and Pressure, and the Master's Secret)

T HE PACE, PRESSURE, and demands of modern life are affecting our ability to be present and attentive, to just relax, listen, and breathe. The effect of life's hectic pace on us is physical, mental, and in some cases, spiritual. We feel it in our marriages, relationships, and careers. It has us at a point where we're feeling that something has got to change, and we're right.

We are all familiar with this definition of insanity:

Insanity is doing the same thing over and over, and expecting a different result.

Individually, and as a society, when we recognize that something isn't working, we attempt to resolve the problem. Sometimes, however, the issues seem too big, or the problems too elusive and we are left not knowing what to do. This feels like one of those times.

Passively and almost unknowingly, we turned away from our intuitive nature, from that quiet voice we used to trust to guide us, the one that rarely lets us down. The noise of life overwhelmed and drowned out our ability to hear that quiet voice and with it our intuitive wisdom. We seem to have lost our compass, doubted or misplaced our connection to our divine and with it the sense of understanding, appreciation, and connection to one another.

Overwhelmed

It has been suggested that people don't care anymore, or that we are either avoiding or unaware of the serious issues. We would rather bury our heads in the sand, in television talent programs, sporting events, and reality shows. Ironically, it's true we are doing that, but it's not because we aren't aware of the serious issues, it's because we are, and we're feeling completely overwhelmed.

Something happens when we become overwhelmed; we go looking for ways to convince ourselves that everything is okay, that life is manageable. We begin to reach for happiness in whatever is closest and most convenient. We pacify ourselves with food, numb ourselves with mood-altering substances, and surround ourselves with more material things than we can afford.

It's a natural reaction; food comforts us, alcohol and other substances relieve stress and make us feel better, at least temporarily, and all the stuff we bought helped us convince ourselves that everything was okay, that life was good. There's just one problem. We all know it isn't working, and to compound the problem, as a society we are now overweight, overly dependent on chemical and liquid pick-me-ups, and often deep in debt.

What Now?

The answer is to begin by taking stock of the good within us, rather than beating ourselves up. Our reaction to the intensity of modern life just reminded us that we're human; we were, and still are, trying to convince our families and ourselves that everything is okay, even if we don't believe it. We are just trying to live our lives and be happy.

Solace

We may find some solace in knowing that this has been going on in societies for as far back as we can remember, but there is something very unique about us and this particular point in history. We are the crest of a wave, that point where the wave has reached its peak, just before it folds over and crashes to the shore. Our actions, like the water of that wave spreading out upon the sand, will carry the message of the course we choose and the results which follow.

Destined for Their Time

It has been suggested that certain individuals are born into their time, from ancient times to the modern day. Plato, Aristotle, Benjamin Franklin, Thomas Jefferson, Abraham Lincoln, Ralph Waldo Emerson, Mahatma Gandhi, Martin Luther King Jr., and even Bill Gates and Steve Jobs all appear to have born into the time that needed them the most.

When the circumstances require it, someone always comes forth with the information that's needed, whether it's to serve a specific need or to advance a society. We believe that the information which we are about to reveal in this book benefits us all individually, and yet also helps us to understand that we are all connected energetically in the dance of life, in our humanity, and this Moment in time.

In this book, we provide insight into an ancient practice called Qigong, and share with you information about the Master and the system which he is offering to us. The Master's program can help us turn off the noise of life and the chatter of our own minds and enter into the quiet where we can reconnect with our intuitive self and our innate wisdom. This sounds like something which we can all benefit from, especially now.

Finally, when we consider that the Master in our story is allowing this information to leave the temple for the very first time in history, and that this event is occurring right now in our lifetimes, it seems like more than mere coincidence; it seems almost destined for its time.

Revealing the Master's Secret

In the chapters ahead we take you with us into an ancient world; we will go behind the temple walls where the Masters in our story developed and perfected the secret practices we will share. We will reveal some of the "Unspoken Codes" and tell you how these were preserved and passed down from one century to the next for almost three thousand years.

Until a few years ago, this information was never allowed beyond the temple walls. Even within the temple, access to these secret practices had to be earned through years of rigorous training. Once training in these programs began, learning and assimilating the vast amount of information encapsulated in Qigong took many more years of dedicated practice to complete.

The information we are about to share is one of the most practical and beneficial wellness programs ever developed.

We will share with you the experiences and testimonials of numerous groups and individuals who have learned, and who continue to, practice these programs. We will include our personal stories, the story of the Master, and how these very programs restored his broken body to a state of health and vitality which changed both the course of his life and the history of this system.

With the Master's permission, we are extending our hand and inviting you to join us as we enter a secret world of unspoken codes and ancient traditions. Perhaps upon reading this book, you will share our belief that this ancient wisdom is both applicable and needed in our modern world and in our daily lives.

Come with us now and together we will take—A Walk with The Master.

CHAPTER 1

"Something's Happening Here" (A Paradigm Shift)

BUFFALO SPRINGFIELD HAD it right when they said "Something's Happening Here" in the lyrics of their song about the social conditions of America in 1970. Looking back, life in the 1970's seems much simpler than life in America, and the world, today. Something is happening, and it has only just begun.

In science, when an old view or theory is replaced by a new one (based upon new scientific findings) it is called a paradigm shift. Whenever we enter a new paradigm, it requires a period of adjustment. For example, numerous scientists and academics spend their entire careers validating, teaching, and defending the current paradigm. These theories and principles are understood to be true, until a new paradigm enters their world.

When a new paradigm enters the picture, it is generally met with a great deal of resistance, including repeated attacks to disprove it. The Big Bang theory, evolution, economic anthropology, and even social networking were all new paradigms which met with great resistance. Change, however, is the great constant. Change is ever-flowing and unavoidable; we are always changing.

Embracing Change

Generally speaking, we often fear what we do not understand. Change, as a rule, means that we have to adjust to a new situation. We have all experienced this in moving to a new job, a new town, a new school, and so on. Change means that we are on unfamiliar turf, and the unfamiliar is often uncomfortable. At a new job, we are alone among new co-workers. In a new town or school, we have to make new friends. In our old jobs, towns, and schools we were established and comfortable, now everything is new and uncomfortable.

At present, we are shifting from an old paradigm to a new paradigm; from thinking externally, materially, and often finitely, to thinking, believing, and acting internally, intuitively, and with an awareness of the infinite, and the divine. This is a shift in social and human consciousness. We are all in this together. We are all aware that we were, and continue to be, practically killing ourselves just to keep up, trying to get ahead in the external, materially driven paradigm (the invisible bubble which we are in.) That approach wasn't working and we knew it intuitively, we just didn't know how to stop it.

We are not going to wake up tomorrow to see that the whole world has suddenly changed. Change, especially internal change, is gradual. What we will begin to realize with greater and greater clarity is that change *has* come. We will find that how we measure the value of our time, our relationships, and even how we expend our energy towards employment has changed. We will begin to notice that the *quality* of our lives is becoming more important and that the *quantity*; the material aspects of our lives is much less important.

We are entering a new paradigm. It isn't something we get to decide whether to participate in or not;

The new paradigm has begun.

It should be understood that the material aspect of our lives is not going to go away. We are human. We need certain things to survive and once those needs are met we will seek to improve our situation, step by step. When we speak of a more aware sense of social consciousness, we are not talking about selling everything we own and running off to live in the woods, although that may be the choice of some people.

An increased sense of awareness or social consciousness begins simply and subtly, and expands. It includes looking at your neighbor potting flowers or mowing their lawn and suddenly realizing that we are all here together. It is recognizing that we want many of the same things, and that we are connected in many ways on many levels.

An increase in consciousness sees no separation in life; it does not keep score or seek to get even. We are all part of the whole, the one. Not everyone will arrive at this awareness at the same time. Those who cling to a world of separation will never have enough, or feel that life is fair, and even. However, every day is a new day, with one more opportunity to walk in the light or to seek and hide in the darkness and negativity. The choice is ours. This book, and the awareness and joy of the Master's Secret, will help us all as we walk in the light and the awareness of our oneness.

The Five Thousand Year Cycle

It has been suggested that periods of consciousness last for five thousand years. This belief is reflected in the predictions of the Mayan calendar. Some believe that The Mayan calendar embodies a prediction of the end of times or the end of human civilization. This belief is causing a great deal of social dialogue and a considerable amount of fear.

We do not believe that the Mayan calendar speaks about, nor that it is predicting, the end of the human race. The human race has gone through many periods of change over the course of history, and it most surely will go through many more. Change is constant; it occurs within and around us every second of every day. We do believe that through given periods of time there is a prevailing foundational or fundamental consciousness, and that this prevailing consciousness, like scientific paradigms, experiences changes from time to time.

If the changes the Mayan calendar speaks of are related to a shift in foundational consciousness, then we would agree that a shift in social consciousness is either taking root or is already underway. As a society, our perspective is shifting away from an external view focused on separateness toward an internal view focused on our connectedness to everything else within the web of creation; the global community, the eco-sphere, and all life on earth.

With this book, we share with you the secret programs which a great Master shared with us. These programs are designed to help us turn down, or turn off, both the noise of the external world and the constant chatter of our own minds. When we do this, we enter the quiet where we reconnect with our own intuitive wisdom and feel the presence and the guidance of our personal divine.

This connection is the key to our internal compass; our personal, intuitive, and enlightened guidance system. When we lose this connection, we feel that our efforts do not match the results we hoped for. We feel detached, disconnected, out of balance, and separated. We feel that the energy flow that once guided us and gave us balance is missing.

It is our sincere hope that by sharing the ancient wisdom embodied in the Master's once secret Qigong your life will be fuller, happier, longer, and filled with greater unity and joy.

CHAPTER 2

The Master's Story—Grand Master Henry Poo Yee (Plus the Opera Singer and More)

BORN IN THE United States, Henry Poo Yee went to China to live with his grandmother at a young age. Returning from China to New York's Chinatown at age fifteen, Master Henry Poo Yee's English was extremely limited. With great determination, he graduated from high school, attended college, and completed a BS in Engineering. Building upon his previous experience in the food service industry, he was soon an owner and partner in restaurants and supper clubs. Returning early one morning from New Jersey to New York, Master Yee was involved in a devastating car accident. He was hospitalized for a long period of time, which included considerable physical therapy and rehabilitation.

At the conclusion of his therapy, the doctors arrived at a shocking prognosis. His hand, which was locked in the shape of a claw, was not going to improve. The damage to the muscle and nerves was too severe to expect further improvement; he would have to go through life in this condition. The worst news, however, was still coming. The doctors determined that the circulation to his leg was not going to improve and amputation was required from the knee down.

A few months earlier, the future Master had been a very successful businessman and college graduate with a bright and promising future. In addition to the devastating news from his doctors, other aspects of his life underwent drastic changes while he was hospitalized. The future Master made a bold decision. He checked himself out of the hospital, financially provided for his family, and flew to Taiwan to see his Master, Lum Sang See. Upon seeing his once promising student arrive at his door, physically crippled and nearly defeated, the Grand Master was moved to tears.

The next morning rehabilitation began. Herbs were gathered from the market; and visits to the nearby country, and a regime of Qigong commenced. At the end of his rehab with Grand Master Lum Sang See, the future Master's hand was relaxed and open and had returned to normal strength. His leg, which the doctors all agreed needed to be amputated below the knee, was also returned to a completely healthy and functioning state.

The Price Tag

Before the Grand Master began treating Poo Yee, his dedicated, long-time student, there was a discussion. If the Grand Master was going to heal his student, he had a request; his student must agree to learn all the Ting Sing Qigong system. Not only must he agree to learn it, he had to agree to carry it on, teach it and ensure that the secrets were not lost. Poo Yee, the future Master agreed.

A New Direction in Life

With any decision we make, the direction of our lives may change considerably. The decision to leave New York and travel to seek the assistance of his Sifu was such a decision for the man who is now the Grand Master of our system. A year earlier he was a successful, up-and-coming club and restaurant owner and family man with businesses in New York and New Jersey. Now he was living with his Sifu in Taiwan and had agreed to teach and represent the Master's system. Few of us will ever go through a change that drastic within our own lifetimes.

The Opera Singer

Decades ago in China, there lived a very successful performer of plays and Chinese Operas. There was, however, a condition which threatened not only her career, but her life; her kidneys were beginning to fail. Initially, the problem only showed in one kidney, which she had removed. The remaining kidney appeared to be in good health and her career resumed for a while, but when that kidney began to show signs of trouble, the situation became dire.

The hospital where she had the first kidney removed had done everything they knew to aid the failing kidney, but nothing worked. She then sought the assistance of hospitals known for alternative natural treatments, but these efforts did not provide the results everyone had hoped for. With her condition deteriorating, it was time to think outside the box. Was there anyone with a non-traditional approach capable of helping her?

Grand Master Lum Sang Sees name came up in these conversations and preparations were made to meet with him. The meeting took place, the terms were agreed to, and the Qigong training began. As a result, her kidney not only returned to its original healthy state, tests indicated that the kidney was larger and healthier than before it began to fail. In those days in China, it was well known that if someone saved your life, you were committed to serving that person for a number of years out of respect and gratitude.

This famous performer did not want to spend the best years of her career in servitude so she chose an alternate route, an acceptable course of action at that time; she paid someone to serve as a personal assistant to Grand Master Lum Sang See in her place.

History Repeats Itself (Sort Of)

In the first six months of the Floating Monk teacher training, Mark Armstrong, OMD, a well-established and highly respected acupuncturist and wellness expert from Atlanta, came to class looking concerned about something.

"Does this system have something to help people with kidney problems?" he asked. "I have a client who brought her adult daughter to me the other day," he said, "the daughter's skin looked like ash, she appeared very ill." He then reported that she had just been told by her doctors that she should go home and prepare to die.

She had been on dialysis, but it was no longer helping very much her kidneys were very weak. She had been on the list for a transplant, but was considered too weak to recover in her current condition. I told Dr Mark that Qigong did have something which may be able to help her; I told him the story of the opera singer.

I showed D Mark the movements most likely to assist this woman, including Chi River Washing, which includes both an internal and an external way to help the body cleanse the kidneys (and other organs) and deliver fresh, more oxygenated blood to those areas. He taught the woman the Qigong which I prescribed. In addition to practicing Qigong, she replaced her old, worn catheter with a new catheter, (the device where the dialysis tubes attach to the body).

Her body responded quickly and positively to the new catheter and the Qigong program which she did at various times throughout the day. She began to do Qigong while she was hooked up to the dialysis machine, and asked those around her to respect her silence as she practiced. Previously, it was reported both the patients and the staff were engaged in gossip and loud conversations on a variety of topics that would fill the room for all to hear. In addition, comfort foods like doughnuts and cookies were frequently brought and shared amongst the group.

Sometimes it is better to light a single candle than to curse the darkness, and this proved to be profoundly true in this case. What began as a simple request for quiet as she practiced her Qigong, and the dialysis machine filtered her blood, soon became much more. To the notice of staff and patients alike, her condition was steadily improving.

Some of the other patients were now asking if they could sit next to her and copy what she was doing, and she agreed. The loud conversations and the unhealthy gossip which once filled the room steadily faded and were replaced by conversations about getting better, how the patients looked better than they had weeks and months before. Her doctors, who had sent her home to die just months before, were now suggesting that her condition was so improved they may even be able to take her off the list for kidney recipients.

There is no clear way of determining how great a role the new catheter or Qigong played in her improved condition. All that is known is that her condition improved to a remarkable degree. There is one other element to consider in her improved health and that is her attitude; her faith, hope, and belief that she was going to get better also played an important role in her marked improvement. Her spiritual faith and the strength she drew from it should also be considered in her journey—from being told to go home and prepare to die, to the vastly improved and hopeful condition which she is in today.

We do not make any claims about Qigong's ability to assist people with serious medical conditions or life-threatening illnesses, but we do stand by the validity of the stories we share with you. Furthermore, we are very careful to ensure that any statement we make is backed by research, is something we have experienced or witnessed first-hand, or comes from a source we know and consider to be above reproach.

CHAPTER 3

Sifu Jim's Story

Sifu Jim's Story

I TURNED SIXTY-FIVE last year. That's quite a milestone in someone's life. It has been quite a journey needless to say. In looking back, I came to the conclusion that there were a few things that really impacted me in monumental ways. One of those is the martial arts. Martial arts practice has changed my life in very significant ways and continues to change my life in many wonderful and different ways.

I find in looking back over this path, what I was looking for and what I found were two different but interrelated things. I learned how to defend myself to feel more secure in a changing world, to be comfortable with myself and the world around me, and to let my guard down and trust life. Most importantly, I learned that we have an inner guidance system that will never let us down if we learn to be still and listen to the wisdom within each and every one of us.

My journey began in 1946 in Marietta, Georgia. The second son of a banker named Bill and a kindergarten teacher named Sadie, I was a sickly child in the beginning but grew out of it quickly. Growing up, all the children in the neighborhood were older and bigger, and some of them were bullies that focused their attention on me. I learned to run fast and throw rocks to get around the problem. It helped some but not enough. What I really wanted to do was learn how to fight. I wanted to be able to pummel those guys and get even big-time. Little did I realize where this desire would lead.

When I was in my teens, I heard about a man who was teaching karate in an old warehouse in my hometown. I went with a friend of mine to check it out and find out first-hand what all the excitement was about. We walked in and I saw this thin red-haired man in a white uniform with the blackest belt I had ever seen. I was hooked the minute I saw him standing there. We watched the class for a little while and then we left. I realized I had found what I was looking for but didn't act on that passion until five years later. By that time I was married and had a wife and family and a full-time job.

I was twenty when I married, and soon after my wife and I had a child on the way. Several years later, we had another child. In the span of five years we had two children, a home, jobs, and a lot of expenses. I began feeling a lot of anxiety at the time and needed some relief.

One day while reading the local paper, I found an article about a karate class starting the following week. I decided to act, believing it might help with the stress. The next day I enrolled in my first Okinawan-style karate class. I loved it, but unfortunately, the anxiety continued to be a problem so I decided to see a counselor. The first visit, he told me changing the way I breathed would help alleviate the anxiety. He went on to explain that when we're stressed our breathing tends to be shallow which only adds to more stress and anxiety. I had learned about the benefits of breathing in karate class but wasn't sold on the idea of it helping with the problems I faced. I didn't pay a whole lot of attention to him at the time and decided he wasn't who I needed to help solve my problems. I continued working, going to karate class, and going through the motions of life. Then I discovered alcohol relieved the anxiety.

I had found a solution or so it seemed. The solution worked for many years until it didn't work anymore. Then I had two problems: alcoholism and anxiety panic disorder. The problem became unbearable and I finally landed in the hospital for treatment of alcoholism. In the hospital, I learned a little about the disease of alcoholism and anxiety panic disorder. Six days later I was released and began attending recovery meetings. I also entered counseling for the panic disorder. That was over twenty-three years ago. I found a solution for the malady that tortured me over the years. The journey has been interesting and oh so wonderful, to say the least. The last twenty-three years have undoubtedly been the very best of my life so far.

When I went into detox, I had lost everything dear to me: Wife, children, career, and possessions. Today my Wife and I are still married after forty-five years. I've reunited with my children and have become a granddad five times over. I do not need to say any more about all the blessings that have come into my life.

When I got out of the hospital, I threw myself into life, but I still had the desire to begin training again in martial arts. Over the years, I had trained in a number of styles and disciplines: Okinawan, Korean, Japanese, and Chinese. I longed to find one style that I really could enjoy and be in long-term. Providence stepped in. A business client was an owner and instructor at a local karate school. He kept after me to come visit him and take a class.

I finally took him up on his offer and in my early forties I began training with Grandmaster Kwan Jo Choi, the founder of Choi Kwang Do International. My Wife began training as well. We both earned the rank of second-degree black belt and rank of chief instructor over the ensuing years. Later we opened a school in our hometown. We had fifteen assistant instructors and over 125 students. A lot of those students went on to become black belts and start schools of their own.

We sold the school in the early 1990s to one of our students. We agreed to stay on and continued to teach. My interests began to shift toward the healing aspects of martial arts. I began studying the various forms of healing, breath therapy, laying on of hands, Reiki, energy healing, pranic healing, and Qigong. During this time I met Dorothy Spitler and Walter Weston, spiritual healers.

I studied under each one for a number of years and was trained in energy healing, spiritual healing, emotional relief therapy, distance healing, and the laying on of hands. While studying with Walter and Dorothy, I came to believe that healing and individual growth and development were my calling. I acted on this insight and enrolled in Coach University and began a two-year program to become a personal coach. While I was learning the new craft of coaching, to earn a living, I reactivated my real estate license and became an associate broker for a local real estate firm specializing in land sales. I worked with developers in an around the Atlanta area in site selection for residential development.

Then fate stepped in. My nephew was one of my students at our old school but had left to pursue another style. At a family gathering, he started telling me about a Kung Fu and Qigong school he was attending. I was again struck with the old desire to learn more. I asked for the instructor's telephone number and I called him the next day regarding Qigong classes. That is how Sifu Jeff and I first met. My Wife and I scheduled an appointment and went to his home for our first lesson. That was in 1995 and we've been learning and training ever since. I haven't missed a day of training in all these years.

The benefits speak for themselves. Prior to beginning a Qigong practice, I had a stiff back every morning. I carried that stiffness with me a good portion of the day. I was in my doctor's office regularly for adjustments. Here's the change that occurred during the first several weeks of practice: I WASN'T STIFF ANYMORE. My body was much more relaxed after Qigong and I felt more energized. Now I know what some of you are thinking, mind over matter. Could be, but it works every day and has for the last seventeen years.

Prior to beginning practice, I was diagnosed with plantar warts about half the size of a golf ball on the bottom of each foot. These rascals were on the ligaments that run from the big toe to the heel. My doctor told me that eventually I would need surgery but that I should wait as long as possible because once they were removed, I would have to stay off my feet for a month or more. I certainly wasn't looking forward to that anytime soon.

I lost myself in life and didn't think about the condition much except when they hurt from too much walking or hiking. Life went on until one day, about nine months later; I noticed that the warts were gone. They had just vanished and haven't come back. The only thing that I did differently was my daily program of Qigong. The results speak for themselves.

The individuals I've worked with have experienced many positive results from Qigong practice, including less stress, more energy, a healthier constitution, less illness, better balance, and heightened awareness. I hope to continue with my Qigong for the next thirty years.

I have remained successful in recovery all these years and have continued working in real estate. I have continued coaching and working with clients from all walks of life both personally and professionally. I have integrated all the training modalities I've learned over the last twenty years into what I like to call transitional coaching: a process that unites the individual with their inner wisdom through the power of the breath.

As I said before, the results speak for themselves.

CHAPTER 4

Sifu Jeff's Story

I GREW UP in small towns in Southern Minnesota. My parents Don and Eleanor Larson had thirteen children, I am number four. My brothers, Kevin and Matt, have gone on ahead. We all miss them very much, and look forward to seeing them again. I attended Catholic grade school in Wabasha and Waseca, and public school in Lake City, where I graduated high school. For a couple of years during high school, our family moved to a suburb of Rockford, Illinois called Loves Park where I attended Harlem High School. I was interested in martial arts from a young age, and was a big fan of the television show Kung Fu with David Carradine, and a big fan of Bruce Lee.

When I moved to Minneapolis following high school, I decided it was time to pursue my interest and began visiting Kung Fu schools. I settled on a system called Southern Praying Mantis. That was almost thirty-five years ago and I am still involved with that system. After seven years in the system, I moved to Atlanta. When I announced that I would be moving to Atlanta, I was told, not asked, that I would be teaching once I got there.

Fate

Once I got settled in Atlanta, I began offering self-defense workshops. My first groups of students were waitresses from the restaurant where I worked, as well as their sisters and friends. By 1987 I had a room at a boxing gym dedicated to Kung Fu; I even sublet the space to another teacher on days when I wasn't teaching. One day a student came in for a private class carrying a flyer for Kung Fu classes just a mile or so from where I was located. Competition from other schools is not unusual, what was unusual was that the system being advertised was the same one I was teaching.

To my knowledge, I was the only person in the South-East teaching this type of Kung Fu, so I was intrigued and went to meet the teacher. Within a few minutes of introducing myself and sitting down to talk with the instructor, I realized that I was in way over my head. I did not know it when I came into the school, but I was in the presence of a Master. I informed my students of the meeting and within a few weeks I closed my school at the boxing gym and we all went to train with the Master.

Looking Back

I have looked back at that day many times over the years and have considered everything that had to take place in order for that meeting to occur. Some people believe in fate, destiny, and serendipity, and others do not. For my part, I believe that my move to Atlanta was predestined. I believe that I was meant to go to Atlanta to meet the Master.

My passion for Qigong and dedication to the system and the Master changed the course of my life. It is that dedication which has driven me for the past twenty-five years. My faith and conviction to Qigong is what pushed me to seek the Master's permission to show this Qigong to the world. That conviction was the driving force in developing Floating Monk. It was the fuel which sustained me over the course of many years as I wrote down, developed, taught, deconstructed, and reconstructed the programs.

As in any journey of this nature, there were sacrifices to be made. The pressure and demands of choosing this path can and did test my conviction and dedication, and it has humbled me repeatedly in the process. Over these many years, there were a number of times when I wanted to walk away; I felt that the demands were too great and the price too steep to continue. Sometimes in life, something grips you so deeply, attaches itself so completely that there is no way to separate yourself from it. When, and if, that happens, it is as if you have no choice, as if fate has found you and the ship has set sail. The destination remains unknown, but the course is set, there is no going back.

Getting Close to the Flame

In Qigong and Kung Fu, we refer to the opportunity to train with the Master as Standing Close to the Flame. The Master is the living body and soul of the system, and very few people have the opportunity to train with a Master directly, especially for an extended period of time. This principle of standing close to the flame can apply to other areas of life as well; sports, business, medicine, entertainment, working with a great chef, or in any number of other fields. If you have the opportunity in your life to stand close to the flame, to feel the pulse, energy, or essence of the knowledge you seek, do so, and savor the experience for it may never come again.

Train at the School, Learn at the Table

Train at the School, Learn at the Table is a term we often refer to in our system. In the school, as one imagines, the training is constant, physically and mentally demanding, and performed under the watchful eye of the Master. In the school, much of the talk is about the forms and techniques different groups and individuals are practicing based on their level; there is not much time for conversation about anything except the training.

Once the evening of training is done, the Master often goes out for dinner. If you are lucky, the Master may invite you to join him for dinner. Once you have been to dinner with the Master, you realize that the discussions there are where the real education takes place. It is there at the table that you learn about the history of the system, hear the stories of long ago, learn about the skills of the Masters that preceded the current Master, and if the opportunity presents itself, you may even be allowed to ask questions. We make a point here about being allowed to ask questions because we often joke (but are actually serious) that there are only two words you need to know to learn Kung Fu and they are: "Yes, Sifu."

The more often you are allowed to dine with the Master, the luckier you are. If you were at the table for many years, you would begin to hear the stories retold, often more than once, and this is no small blessing. In hearing the stories retold, you hear parts you had forgotten or perhaps missed on the first, second, or tenth telling. After hearing the stories told a couple of times (due to new people being invited to the table) you had a pretty good grasp. I was very fortunate when I closed my school and came with my students to train under the Master, as he allowed me to be his assistant instructor. This position allowed me to join the Master almost every evening for dinner. I now tell my students the stories which the Master told me all those years ago.

Our First International Tournament

In the autumn of 1991, the Master and I attended an international martial arts tournament in Houston, Texas. I went to compete and the Master went to teach workshops and see old friends. I competed in the Qigong division Internal Arts. When you complete your routine, you salute and stand at attention awaiting your score. As I finished my program, I could see the three judges in the center and far corners of the ring looking at one other. I noticed the same thing occurring with the corner judges to my left and right. They flipped the numbers on their cards and I soon saw the 9.9 and 9.8 scores appearing from the five judges. I knew I was near the top. One by one the other competitor's entered and exited the ring. As soon as the competition was finished, the scores were announced. At the very first tournament that the Master's Qigong was seen, it won the gold medal.

I ran upstairs and waited for Sifu to notice me in the room where he was teaching a workshop. I told him that I'd won the gold medal; that was one of the proudest Moments of my life. Although I was happy for myself, I was even happier for my Sifu as the gold medal was a clear statement of what the other Masters thought of Sifu's Qigong and Kung Fu. Sifu left Atlanta and moved to Houston a few months after the tournament. The following year in 1992, I attended the same tournament, this time held in Orlando, Florida. I went with students Sapir Tal, now Sifu Sapir Tal who is living and teaching in Israel, and Luis Cardozo, now living in Uruguay. I was extremely pleased with the results as each of them left the competition with gold and silver medals.

Before returning to college a few years later, I competed in a South-East regional tournament with other members of the Atlanta Branch School lead by Sifu Peter Goulburne and assistant instructors John Hall and Jonathan Gass. Once again, the Master's Qigong took home the gold medal and every member of the Atlanta School left the tournament with two or three medals. Peter took the helm of the Atlanta Branch School just before the tournament, and I turned to teaching private students while attending college full-time and working part-time. That was almost seventeen years ago. It is amazing how time flies.

After completing my BA in Finance in 1999, I began a new career in financial services. In March of 2011, I completed my MBA and now spend my time between the two worlds of finance and Qigong. I believe that in time the financial services I provide will find a place alongside other services (under the Floating Monk umbrella) which focus on the quality of our lives.

CHAPTER 5

Understanding what Chi is and the Origins of Qigong

Q IGONG, (PRONOUNCED *CHEE kung*) is also called Chi Kung in North America and many European countries. There are additional ways of writing or pronouncing Qigong, but the meaning is the same; they all refer to breathing practices which are credited with improving health, increasing our life energy and life expectancy, as well as promoting the healing of ailments or injuries. As a general rule, Qigong programs are done either sitting or standing and often include a series of gentle, flowing movements.

The Translation of the word Qigong is this: *qi* (or *chi*) means "breath" and *gong* (or *kung*) means "work." These words also have a deeper meaning: *chi* means energy or life force, and *gong* (or *kung*) means an advanced practice.

Qigong may also be described as:

A method for increasing, storing, and focusing your life energy

The reason there are so many stories about Qigong achieving amazing results is that Qigong deals directly with your life force, your chi. By using your breath, body postures, and gentle, flowing movements perfected over many centuries, these programs circulate your life force, your chi, throughout your body. As your chi circulates, it removes blockages allowing your energy, your life force, to flow properly. The next step is to increase and store even more chi and then learn to focus this energy towards your goals and visions for life. The results and benefits are as varied as the programs being offered. For this reason it is important to verify the credentials of both the program and the instructor. Read more on this in the section The Unspoken Codes.

Where the Secrets Began

Prior to sharing the Master's gift, it is important to have at least a basic understanding of where Qigong comes from, how it evolved, and why this Master's information remained a secret for all these years. We will provide the following brief history of Qigong prior to discussing the Master's secret. Later in the book, we will provide a more detailed history of the Master's System, including how he formed the first new branch from the original system. We will also explain how Floating Monk followed the Master's example and became the first new branch from his lineage.

In the Beginning: The Ancient Caves

The earliest records of Qigong date back about six thousand years to caves along the Yangtze River in China. In these caves are wall drawings of bodies performing what appear to be a connected and flowing series of movements similar to the movements used in Qigong. There is no information available about these drawings, yet experts suggest they are the earliest known depictions of Qigong.

The Yellow Emperor: The Birth of Chinese Medicine and Qigong

The most conclusive documented information on Qigong takes us back to the time of the Yellow Emperor Gongsun. The period of The Yellow Emperor in China extends from 2,697 to 2,967 BC. The Yellow Emperor is credited with the formal introduction of traditional Chinese medicine, as well as the first recorded material on Qigong.

"If you want to live to be one hundred, do Qigong."

Dr. Oz

From the Two Schools to the World

Generally speaking, after the time of The Yellow Emperor, Qigong practices developed and grew forth from two different sources or schools: Taoist and Buddhist (Shaolin). The Taoist temples produced numerous Qigong programs as well as the popular exercise known as Tai Chi. Likewise;

the Buddhist (Shaolin) temples also produced many powerful Qigong programs, but are more readily known for bringing us Kung Fu.

Northern and Southern China

Martial arts and Qigong systems often define themselves as being northern or southern, meaning from northern or southern China. The movements of the northern systems tend to be wide and sweeping and take more room to perform. The southern systems tend to have shorter, more compact motions and favor close-range contact. Geography helps us to understand the reason for this as the North has sweeping plains and more open spaces, while the South is characterized by bamboo forests and more confined terrain. Taoist systems are often viewed as northern and Buddhist (Shaolin) systems as southern, although this is by no means a hard and fast rule.

Our Programs

The programs we are about to share with you operate from a fundamental belief that all of us have a personal life force, or personal energy. This energy, for over three thousand years, has been called chi. Our programs teach you to move this energy, or chi, throughout your body to reduce stress, relax your mind and body, enhance your circulation, cleanse and strengthen your internal organs (your engine) and provide you with more energy than you've probably felt for many, many years.

Qigong as Medicine

For thousands of years, specialized breathing programs were one of the primary tools of traditional Chinese medicine. These specialized breathing programs were developed over the course of many centuries. Many Shaolin and Taoist monks dedicated their entire lives to developing and perfecting these programs. These specialized programs were referred to as Qigong and those who perfected these systems were known as Qigong Masters.

> "Qigong can help us stretch and stay loose and balance both mind and body. It allows us to cope with the day to day struggles of being human."
>
> **Dr. Oz**

The Fountain of Youth

Over the centuries Qigong has been referred to in many ways: the fountain of youth, the breath of life, the secret elixir, the practice of the three treasures, and many other names. Certain, advanced Qigong programs, teach practitioners to make their bodies conduits between earth and heaven by first drawing the energy into themselves, and then releasing the energy back to its source.

Some of these programs have been preserved over the centuries, some have been lost forever, and others, like the Qigong in this book, had never been allowed to leave the temple, remaining a secret for all these years.

Their Secret Weapon: Chi

The specialized breathing programs (Qigong programs) developed and practiced in ancient Chinese temples have slowly come to public knowledge over the course of many centuries. For time immemorial, it has been rumored that the monks in these temples, and many of the legendary warriors in Chinese folklore, had developed special powers through the practice of Qigong, in other words, that Qigong was somehow their secret weapon.

The Master: Passing on the System

In this book we explain to the reader a set of simple, yet very unique programs which can increase energy, advance awareness, improve health, and perhaps even prolong life. These secret programs were passed down from a great Master to his inner circle of long-time disciples called the Enter the Gate Disciples.

The fact that the Master is allowing us to share this gift with the public at a time when it is so needed is more than a simple gesture of kindness;

It is an act of love.

Our Thoughts and Our Energy

Wherever we direct our thoughts and our attention, we are also directing our energy. Our thoughts are energy and the actions we take are expressions of that energy. We intuitively understand this when we say "I have a lot of energy today" or "the energy in the room was really good." This idea, which seems profound, is actually something we not only understand, but refer to throughout our day. When quantum physics proclaimed that "everything is energy" it didn't come as news to us, we (as a society) already knew this.

The simple daily programs we present in this book, which appear to be a new way of approaching and energizing your day, are not new at all; these programs are the pearls of ancient wisdom. These enjoyable, easy-to-perform programs of relaxed breathing and gentle movement that help to increase, store, and manifest our energy date back thousands of years. They have been practiced, preserved, and passed down from one Master to the next this entire time.

Energy: the Alpha and the Omega

We use the word energy frequently throughout this book, primarily as it refers to your energy, the energy within you, and the universal energy that surrounds you. The programs, which we will reveal and discuss, will tell you how to increase, store, and manifest your energy towards the powerful and attainable vision you have for your life.

With the Master's permission, we invite you to join us as we enter a secret world of unspoken codes and ancient traditions.

This ancient wisdom is both applicable and needed in our modern world, and our daily lives. Come with us now and together we will take . . .

A walk with the Master

CHAPTER 6

Understanding a Pai when
Math meets Mystery

Both Halves of the Circle

A S WE PULL back the curtain and begin to reveal the structure, practices, and principles of the ancient temples, we first need to tell you what a pai is. This will give you the ability to look at any program and accurately define whether the program is a pai, a style, or simply information that was gathered and put together to develop a specific type of program.

For me, as a long-time practitioner of a very traditional temple-based system, I ardently believe in teachers being up-front, honest, and willing to share with students the origins and validity of any program they are offering.

As Qigong grows in popularity, which it will for many years to come, there are those in our society who will see Qigong as an opportunity to enrich themselves, in short,

The Charlatans are coming.

There are few things that disturb us more than dishonesty. If someone has dedicated themselves to a noble and true practice, put in the time, worked hard and learned a program, then by all means they have earned the right to represent that program in the public arena.

We firmly hold that every program being offered to the public should meet specific criteria. The minimum requirement should be to clearly define the source of the information, such as we have done by providing the history of our program and identifying every Master up to the present day. We also believe that adherence to the Unspoken Codes is part of this requirement as it asks the question; "Who's Your Sifu?" and allows the student to determine if the Sifu (teacher) Reflects the Light.

In traditional Qigong the teacher (Sifu) is a messenger, a reflection of the light. The Sifu is a reflection of original system and the Master's that came before them. When the role of a teacher is viewed in this way, it is extremely important that the teacher's actions honor the linage of their system.

A Pai, a System, or a Program

In the Qigong (and Kung Fu) world there two main descriptors: 1) a complete system or pai, and 2) a style. In the past few decades a third term has emerged: a program.

A pai refers to a complete system. A complete system has two halves, like the two halves of a circle. One half is made up of forms, fighting, and weapons; the other half is medicine, healing, and Qigong. The Master of a pai often excels in other areas as well, such as calligraphy, philosophy, poetry, painting and other such disciplines which we in Western civilization refer to as the arts and letters.

These two halves serve to balance each other. If you learn to kill, you must learn to heal. If you learn to strike, you must learn to yield. If you condition your bones to be like steel, you must also be able to flow like water. The symbol of yin and yang, the balance between both halves, is symbolic of a complete system or pai. In order to have a pai, it is necessary to have a Master. We do not mean someone who has mastered a system or a practice, we mean the Master of the system.

A style is not a complete system; a style reflects pieces of a complete system. As a general rule, a style is designed specifically for fighting. A style does not teach a complete program, it is a piece of a program, or a piece of a pai. Many of the martial arts schools in North America and Europe today are styles.

In ancient times there was no such thing as a police force. In those days the wealthy families in towns and villages, and occasionally the villagers themselves, paid accomplished martial artists to teach them self-defense.

This was accurately depicted in the movie *The Seven Samurai*. These martial artists taught the townspeople and villagers the easiest, most direct and lethal techniques they knew, including open hand and weapons techniques, which they gleaned from the martial arts system they had trained in. Many of the styles which are popular today actually originated in this way.

A program is neither a pai (a Complete System) nor a style (a piece of a Complete System). Programs are often developed using pieces of information from a variety of sources. At other times, programs were developed using a single idea or practice from a pai, a style, or even from another program.

Numerous self-help programs, as well as many modern practitioners using titles like energy worker, energy healer, and energy guide and other such titles do not provide any specific historical source as the foundation of their training, understanding, or skill.

Others claim to have information from, or a connection to, a wide variety of sources. Having information from a wide variety of source can be a good thing, but we believe that the practitioner offering services to the public owes it to them to identify these sources as well as the level of understanding, training, and certification they have achieved.

The American Indian culture is an excellent example of identifying the source of their knowledge and the level of their understanding. In the American Indian culture the practitioner, shaman, or medicine man always identifies their tribe, their teacher, and their level of understanding. This kind of openness and honesty not only respects the source of their knowledge as well as the grandfathers and the Great Spirit, it also demonstrates a respect for the person coming to them for treatment or healing.

Identifying the source and showing a respect for the system, the teacher, the tribe, and the culture is of vital importance. It is this acknowledgement which helps to create the connection to the spirits, Great Spirit (American Indian) or the Masters and the Universe (Chinese) whose help, energy, and guidance the healer is seeking to transfer to the person who has come to them.

We prefer to believe that every individual, and all of the groups that are currently offering services in the public marketplace, are sincere in their efforts and that their intentions are good. As for our organization, we know what we offer and we speak about what we know. It is not our place to speak to the validity of other programs, but we would offer this piece of advice: the Unspoken Codes can be applied to any program, and the answers you receive should provide the information you need to make an informed decision.

Math and Mystery

In the ancient temples, Qigong programs were developed and perfected within the framework of a complete system or pai. As we mentioned, a pai is symbolized by a circle, with two equal and perfectly balanced halves. Balance was the objective; life was the journey or the process.

From the early days of mathematics, pi symbolized as π (equaling 3.14159) is a mathematical constant that is the ratio of a circle's circumference. Because the definition of pi relates to the circle, pi is found in many disciplines such as trigonometry, geometry, mechanics, and electromagnetism. The further one advances into Qigong (and the martial arts) the more you see and understand the theory and application of geometry and physics. With enough time, you will come to see movement in terms of geometric or mathematical shapes and formulas. Like the circle, the further you get from the source, the closer you get to the beginning.

In the later, more advanced stages of Qigong practice, quantum physics becomes more and more relevant, especially in describing what is happening in terms of energy. This may sound complex, but it isn't, it is as logical as it is simple. As Sifu Jim noted in his comments from Einstein: "everything is energy." When energy is blocked, we feel uncomfortable, frustrated and out of balance. When energy is flowing, we feel light, energetic and in balance. We use terms like this every day, so the discussion of energy is not foreign to us at all. We just didn't realize how smart we were, we have been talking in terms of quantum physics our entire lives.

Ancient and Modern

From Ancient Greece we received the formula pi "π," and from ancient China we received the term pai, represented by the yin-yang symbol. Both pi and pai refer to circles, both are constants; they are unwavering. Both of these symbols serve as foundations. Pi "π" serves as a foundation for mathematics, mechanics, engineering and more. Pai, represented by yin—yang, serves as the foundation for balance of two separate yet equal and united halves. It speaks to the idea of spirit and body, of internal and external (or inside and outside), of upper and lower, and of body and mind.

Encapsulated within the symbol of yin-yang is the idea we refer to as: As Above-So Below. This idea is interwoven into any definition or explanation of the two halves of the circle. The symbol of yin-yang and the concept of As Above-So Below permeate all of human existence. They serve not only as guidelines for practices within systems; they provide a philosophical foundation for what we do, and how we live our lives. Finally, both symbols remain as relevant today, in the twenty-first century, as they were the Moment they were first conceived.

Qigong is not Tai Chi

Publically there is confusion regarding Qigong and Tai Chi, namely that people often think they refer to the same thing. They do not.

Tai Chi, known formally as Tai Chi Chuan, is a martial art System. It is a product of the Taoist temples or the Taoist school. Tai Chi Chuan means Supreme Ultimate Fist. Tai Chi is widely known as a gentle, slow-moving exercise, which we often see being practiced in public parks, especially early in the mornings.

In reality, Tai Chi Chuan is an extremely powerful and highly effective martial art. There are a number of excellent Tai Chi Masters in the United States and Canada who teach Tai Chi to the full extent of its potential, but there are also a number of teachers who teach Tai Chi as more of a gentle exercise than as a powerful martial art.

Tai Chi Chuan as a system (or pai) does have numerous Qigong programs, many of which are referred to by animal names or as various treasures. These Qigong programs vary widely depending upon the teacher or Master, and the range of the programs which they know (have trained in) and are willing to teach. Perhaps the biggest reason that Qigong and Tai Chi are confused by many people is because they sound similar; both Tai Chi and Qigong have the word chi in them.

Summary

There are many different types of Tai Chi, as well as numerous different systems of martial arts, and many of these programs offer their own unique type of Qigong. The fact that there are so many diverse programs to choose from makes it very difficult for someone to know which to choose.

Keep it Simple

At Floating Monk, we believe that programs should be clear, easy to explain, enjoyable to perform, and that the benefit should be felt as soon as the first class. We also believe that it is vital to be honest with oneself about how long you are willing to practice each day. The majority of our programs are designed as ten to fifteen-minute practices. If a person is rushed, they can do a simple five minute program. On days when a person has more time they can do twenty minutes or more, adding the Stretching Qigong to the Sitting or Standing Qigong for an even more enjoyable and beneficial program.

CHAPTER 7

The Master's System is a pai

THE MASTER WE refer to in this book is Grand Master Henry Poo Yee. Great Grand Master Lum Sang See (his teacher) gave Grand Master Yee the nick name Poo (or Po) in reference to the Last Emperor of China, Po Yi. Perhaps Great Grand Master Lum Sang See had a vision of the legacy which Grand Master Yee would create, and gave him this nickname as a reference to what he would accomplish and the impact his knowledge would have upon the world.

The original system in which Ting Sing Qigong originated is called *Kwongsai Jook Lum Gee Tong Long Pai*. As indicated by its name, it is a complete system, or pai. From its origin in the late 1800s, prominent names associated with the system are Som Dat, Lee Shiem See, Cheung Yel Chung, Lum Sang See, and the current Grand Master Henry Poo Yee. For detailed information on these Masters, as well as more information about the System, visit Grand Master Yee's website CKFA.com and click on History. While you are there, be sure to click on the tab for Grand Master Yee's personal history, we are confident that you will enjoy learning more about him.

Grand Master Yee forms a New Pai

When Grand Master Yee completed his rehabilitation with Great Grand Master Lum Sang See and accepted the responsibilities associated with his new title, he decided to form a new branch from the original tree. This new branch would be the very first pai born out of the original system. Grand Master Yee named this new pai Chinese Kung Fu Academy U.S.A. (CKFA. com). This information is also available on the Grand Master's website.

Floating Monk is born

When Grand Master Yee allowed me to take the Qigong out of the temple and show it to the public for the first time, he made his permission conditional. The name Ting Sing could not be used in the public arena, it had to stay in the temple. For the first few years, I called the Qigong Chi for Health and many people still know it by this name, but the Internet soon revealed that this name was too generic. I did not wish for people attempting to find us via the Internet to get lost in a sea of chi-related queries, so a new name was needed.

In Chinese mythology there were a group of very unique messengers. These messengers were called upon whenever important information needed to get to the Emperor, or between generals who were some distance from one another during great battles and at times of war. It was rumored that these messengers would write special symbols on pieces of paper, adhere the paper to their calves, and that upon doing so they would levitate.

Using the power of their intent, it is said that these monks could travel at great speeds and that if seen from a distance they appeared to be floating. These monks were aptly referred to as the floating monks. We believe that we too are the bearers of important information, because we are bringing the information about this unique Qigong to the public for the first time. It is for this reason that we chose to call our organization Floating Monk and title the Qigong Floating Monk Qigong.

The Unspoken Codes

Behind the temple walls, steeped in ancient tradition are the Unspoken Codes. These codes have guided the behavior of Qigong Sifus and Masters from the earliest days and are as alive today as they were thousands of years ago. When Teachers, Sifus and Masters bring their knowledge to the public arena, other Teachers, Sifus and Masters are watching to see if they are following the codes.

The Inner Circle

Membership in the inner circles of high-level Qigong is steeped in ritual; burning incense, kneeling, saluting, recitations, and a number of other aspects which unfortunately cannot be mentioned here. The details of what occurs during these ceremonies are not what's important, what is important is the commitment to uphold and reflect the integrity of the system, both publicly and privately.

These commitments encapsulate what we refer to as the Codes of Conduct. The uniqueness of the Codes of Conduct is that, in many cases, these codes are embedded into the information provided and the terms which are agreed to, but they are not verbalized. These commitments exist as a type of contract. If you walk a certain path you are expected to abide by this unwritten contract; you are expected to uphold the codes.

The codes are the guidelines for the Sifu's behavior, especially in public, and you never break the codes.

The codes are the links of a chain that connects the Sifu to those that came before him or her, and you never, ever break the chain.

What are the Secret Codes?

It is an unwritten rule that the codes are expected to be maintained by each system that offers its programs to the public, and by the individuals who represent that system. There is no established group for monitoring the codes; they are the guidelines by which a Sifu is to monitor their own behavior. Invisible to the public eye, these codes are the lens through which Instructors, Sifus and Masters observe the public behavior of their peers.

These codes are referred to, almost in passing, during the ceremony, marking your entry into the Inner Gate. In a strange and mysterious way, the fact that some of the codes are mentioned so subtly actually punctuates their importance. When the Master casually talks about what can occur if certain codes are broken, you suddenly realize that the mysteries which you have heard about and wondered about for so many years are actually true. That realization is a powerful and memorable Moment.

The Codes which May be Mentioned

Of all the rules within the codes, there are a few which may be mentioned publicly because they deal with public behavior. In the coming years, as Qigong becomes more and more popular, we believe that it will be beneficial for the public to have some way of understanding and differentiating between various types of programs, including those that do and those that do not follow the codes.

Of the two codes which may be mentioned, the first is known as Reflecting the Light and the second is Who's your Sifu?

The First Code: Reflecting the Light

There is a belief in Chinese culture regarding success: "Be careful about rising too high or too fast because the higher you go, the further you can fall." This idea does not suggest that a person should not try to be successful; rather, it speaks to the idea of being sure-footed, and of building on a sound foundation. Success can be fleeting or it can be long-lasting, and the definition of success varies between individuals, cultures, and nations.

In Qigong, we believe that success begins by giving credit to those responsible for it; including recognizing, naming, and showing gratitude towards that person. Success in Qigong means Reflecting the Light. An ancient tradition, it is one of the most fundamental Unspoken Codes. Historically, it would have been applied the first time that a Master graduated a student and allowed him or her to go out into the world to begin their teaching career. Every time that new teacher received praise, the next words out of his or her mouth should be; thank you, I had a great teacher.

Humility

At the center of Reflecting the Light is humility. True humility is sincere and grateful; it recognizes that your success is owed in part (often in large part) to the time and energy that your teacher has dedicated to you, and the information which they have imparted to you. Yes, you had to do the work, often a great deal of work once you possessed the knowledge, but still, your teacher had to give it to you.

We see reflections of this code within our own society, for example, when a public figure or celebrity speaks about how a certain teacher influenced their life. When they tell stories about how a certain teacher or college professor saw something in them gave them their time and guided them, this is Reflecting the Light. The same principle holds true in Qigong.

There is something innately satisfying about being in the presence of someone who is truly great and sincerely humble. Mahatma Gandhi and Martin Luther King, Jr. were such individuals. Other such persons may include Albert Einstein, Ralph Waldo Emerson, Robert Frost, and based on interviews I have seen, even Quincy Jones. As a society, we tend to have great respect for those who show sincere humility, and in like fashion we tend to abhor those whose egos far exceed their talents or their deeds.

The Codes as Guides

The Codes of Conduct are there to provide a guideline which we can use to see who is Reflecting the Light, and they help to steer us clear of those who Absorb the Light. In Qigong, someone who Reflects the Light always happily gives credit to their Instructor, Sifu, or Master.

When you compliment someone who Reflects the Light, the very next words out of their mouth are always, "thank you, I had great teacher." Likewise, someone who Absorbs the Light will take the credit, mention nothing of their teacher, and wear their knowledge publicly with arrogance and pride.

The Second Code: Who's Your Sifu?

In their entirety, the Codes of Conduct speak to behavior both public and private. Individuals who follow the path the codes outline are inwardly focused on their own behavior; they don't teach the codes or admonish anyone who lives by other guidelines. They simply live their lives by quiet example.

The codes will not be found anywhere in writing. They are never mentioned in the literature about classes, workshops, or in any training manuals. The codes are rarely even discussed outside of the special ceremonies where a Sifu or Master is graduating a student. If you have the opportunity to train with a certified Sifu, you may hear them discuss behavior in general terms from time to time. The onus is on the student to pick up on these subtle suggestions for they are the Sifu's way of giving the student insight into the Unspoken Codes.

Behind the curtain, however, in the world of certified Instructors, Sifus, and Masters, these codes are considered unwritten law. When a teacher introduces themselves, whether it is to another teacher or to a class or workshop, the introduction should always be: "Hello, my name is (their name), I teach (the name of the system) and my Sifu/Master is (Sifu/Master's name)."

The Question Has Three Parts

For someone who is seeking out a Qigong program to study, the codes provide these simple questions. To the question of, Who's your Sifu?, there are three parts that, added together, will provide enough information to let you know if you are speaking with a qualified, certified instructor who follows the codes and Reflects the Light. The three questions are:

1. What system do you teach?
2. Who is your Sifu/Master?
3. What level are you certified to teach?

CHAPTER 8

Behind the Curtain
(The Secret Techniques Revealed)

GRAND MASTER YEE has spent his life training, perfecting, preserving and passing on the Kung Fu of the Chinese Kung Fu Academy U.S.A. and the Ting Sing Qigong which Great Grand Master Lum Sang See taught him.

Without Grand Master Yee's permission, this Qigong would never have been available to the public, and the lives of many people who have benefited from this Qigong would be very different. In addition to our gratitude to Grand Master Yee, we are also thankful to his Sifu, Great Grand Master Lum Sang See, and Great, Great Grand Master Lee Shiem See for developing the original program.

Mensa meets Shaolin and the Tao (A Master like No Other)

The impact that Great, Great Grand Master Lee Shiem See had upon this system was, and remains today, immense. His level of intelligence is displayed in his understanding of the *I Ching* (The Book of Changes), Taoism, Buddhism, astronomy, physics, geometry, electromagnetism, Chinese medicine, nature and the four seasons, and much more. The great Master brought his understanding of all of these areas together in one place, the Qigong Program which he developed and titled Ting Sing Qigong.

Ting Sing, as we have mentioned, means "to make the universe shine." In application, this means to make the energy of the universe shine forth from you, the practitioner. In all the years of training and teaching Qigong and Kung Fu, through local, state, regional and international tournaments, observing numerous Master's demonstrations, and reading a wide array of books and assorted research, I have never seen a Qigong Program that is anything like Lee Sum See's Ting Sing Qigong.

Immediate Benefit

One of the most intriguing aspects of Ting Sing (Floating Monk Qigong) is that the benefits begin as soon as you start to practice. Of course, the more you practice and the better you get at relaxing, breathing, and performing the movements, the more benefit you receive. The movements of this Qigong are simple and easy to understand, and this simplicity allows students to adjust or correct their posture when practicing on their own.

When the teacher tells you what these simple movements and breathing techniques are doing, and you feel the chi inside your body wake up and begin to flow, you start to really enjoy and connect with the Qigong. Once this happens, which is usually very early in Qigong training, you begin to look forward to waking up and practicing your Qigong every day.

A Glimpse inside the Qigong

A simple list of some of the elements which Lee Shiem See includes in this Qigong will help to clarify the depth of his wisdom:

- Stepping Into the Circle
- The Four Directions
- The Two Vortexes
- Finding your Place on the Earth
- The Six Sections of the Circle
- As Above-So Below
- The Three Rings of Chi
- The Four Winds
- The Four Chimneys
- The Four Exits
- Eating from Heaven
- Yin/Yang/Yin
- The Three Gates
- Thunder in the Cave
- The Highest High
- The Empty Force
- The Five Elements
- Washing The Chi River

- Reverse Breathing
- The Zipper
- Opening and Closing the Third Eye

**It wasn't a matter of just being incredibly intelligent;
Lee Shiem See was a genius.**

Stepping Into the Circle

Stepping into the Circle is the technique which begins the Qigong practice. There is a visual component related to this technique, and from the very first Moment on the very first day, this technique lays the foundation for something we call the Conversation with Heaven. Once inside the circle, you begin to adjust your feet; this is the beginning of the Four Directions, which leads to the Twin Vortexes and Finding Your Place on the Earth. This technique is only practiced with the Standing Qigong.

The Three Treasures

The Three Treasures is not an idea unique to Floating Monk; it is part of a broader philosophy. According to Taoist doctrine, the Three Treasures can be described as the three types of energy available to humans. Speaking generally, they are known as Jing, Chi, and Shen.

Jing refers to our human bodies and its abilities. Chi refers to our personal internal energy and our life force. It is important to note that chi is considered to be in all things.

Shen refers to the spirit. Within this context it refers not only to our spirit, for it presupposes that we have a spirit, but to the broader spiritual world beyond and above us. In some Qigong practices it is believed that the practitioner may enter Shen.

The Twin Vortexes

To begin Floating Monk (Standing) Qigong, the practitioner steps Into the Circle, adjust the feet in a prescribed fashion, and begins to circle (rotate the body). To the casual observer, this motion looks very odd, but the Floating Monk practitioner understands this motion is creating what we call the Twin Vortexes. The first vortex draws the energy from the earth upward into the body. The second vortex draws the energy through the body and sends the energy toward heaven, from which it returns.

The more familiar and more comfortable the practitioner gets with this motion; the easier it is to relax and thus flow within the motion. The footwork, including the width of the feet and the movement within the feet, requires that they be positioned correctly. The motions must be properly performed to create the desired effect.

The Four Winds

The Four Winds element introduces itself very early in the Standing Qigong and arises again with greater detail in the more advanced practice. The Four Winds is very prevalent in Level III and Level IV. It refers not only to the four directions, but also to the angle of the hands and arms while performing the movement.

When practicing the Four Winds, if the angles of the hands are correct, the hands will adjust the wrist, the wrist will adjust the elbow, the elbow will adjust the shoulders, and the shoulders will speak to and adjust the body. The entire body will be one, which is flowing with and connected to the energy and movement. If the angles of the wrist are not correct, every other section of the structure will be, what we refer to as, broken. If the structure is broken, the energy will not accumulate or run properly throughout the body.

Yin/Yang/Yin

Yin/Yang/Yin is one of the most profound and yet easily understood concepts of our practice. Yin/Yang/Yin, loosely translated, means soft/hard/soft. The introduction of this theory places us firmly on the doorstep of quantum physics, there's simply no way around it. We mentioned earlier in the book that everything is energy. It is here in Yin/Yang/Yin that the presence of quantum physics becomes clear.

In both Standing and Sitting Qigong, most of the program is done in a relaxed (yin) state. At a specific point towards the end of the exercise (in Sitting Qigong) the practitioner adjusts their hand position in preparation for squeezing the body which is a transition into yang. The practitioner will apply a squeezing motion at a specific point in the breathing cycle, and will perform this yang technique for a specific number of cycles. Following this series of yang squeezes, the practitioner transitions briefly back into a yin state. This practice is known as Yin/Yang/Yin.

Opening and Closing the Physical and Energy Body

When the practitioner is in the yin state, muscles, bones, and tendons are relaxed. The idea is for this relaxation to reach all the way down to the cells of your body. This relaxation allows for the free flow of the energy inside the body. When the body is sufficiently yin (open) the entire body begins to breathe in the air and energy around it. When you transition in yang, you learn to seal in the energy that has entered your body. Upon return to a yin state, you do what we call scanning the body, which sends the mind and breath through the body to search for, speak to, and relax any muscle or organ that might still be tense, or what we call holding.

As Above-So Below

As Above-So Below is a broad idea that refers to matching, repeating, mirroring, and at the same time balancing, that which is on earth with that which is in heaven. It also refers to the upper half and the lower halves of the body.

We mentioned in Yin/Yang/Yin that there were points in the form where you squeeze the body. Applying this concept to the concept of As Above-So Below (in the Standing Qigong) if we squeeze at a given point when the hands are in the upper part of the body, then we must also squeeze when the hands are located at a given point in the lower part of the body.

The Four Chimneys

The Four Chimneys refer to four locations on the body. During the practice of either the Sitting or Standing Qigong, the body creates heat. In the body's effort to disperse or release this heat, it uses the Four Chimneys, which we also refer to as vents.

As the body disperses the heat through these vents, it carries some degree of moisture along with the heat, which we refer to as steam. It is believed that this steam carries with it the impurities that are present in the body. For this reason, we say that as the body releases this steam out of the Four Chimneys, the body is steaming out the poison.

New Qigong practitioners are very often surprised to find that a measurable amount of steam has been released by the body through the Four Chimneys, and yet they did not feel it (or sometimes believe it) until they checked the locations of the Four Chimneys and realized that it had occurred.

Internal and External

It may seem odd to mention the word "external" in the context of describing a Qigong program, after all, isn't Qigong an internal practice? The answer to that question is both yes and no. Yes, Qigong is considered an internal exercise or program because it is primarily a practice of specialized, relaxed breathing techniques; however, there is an external aspect of Qigong as well: the skin.

We often refer to Qigong as a program of health from the inside out, meaning that it focuses on breathing and the health and vitality of the internal organs. Many people are surprised, however, when they are asked to name the largest organ of the body. It is our skin. That's right, our skin is an organ and it is the largest organ of our entire body.

A Complete System and a Complete Qigong

Earlier, we defined what a complete system, or pai, is. Not only are there complete systems in martial arts, there are complete systems in Qigong as well. A complete system in Qigong, as symbolized by the yin-yang symbol, has two parts; internal and external. Sometimes, although it is quite rare, a system may have (as Floating Monk does) a Yin/Yang/Yin component as well.

Washing the Chi River

The external component of Floating Monk Qigong is called washing the Chi River. Between (and within) each of the seven layers of skin, and between the skin and our muscles, is a fluid, referred to in Qigong as the Chi River. The Chi River, it is suggested, becomes polluted with toxins as the body works to filter itself and maintain proper balance.

Chi River Washing uses a special series of techniques to rid the body of the toxins within. This process also helps to reduce naturally occurring stress hormones, such as cortisol. Stress hormones can build up and cause our body's considerable stress-related damage, including heart attacks and stroke. It is important when reviewing various Qigong programs to know if they have a process for Chi River Washing.

The Four Exits

In the process of external cleansing such as washing the Chi River, it is important to consider how the toxins and other impurities are going to get out of the body. This leads to the discussion of the Four Exits. Actually, there are a total of six exits, but the first four are specifically related to the Chi River. It is not enough for a program to suggest that a process or technique helps to cleanse the body; this is the information age and we want to know exactly how the program actually does what it says it can.

CHAPTER 9

The Master's Secret
(Health from the Inside Out)

IN THE PAGES leading up to this chapter, we have mentioned a number of benefits related to the practice of Floating Monk Qigong. It is now time to talk specifically about the Master's secret.

The Master's Secret, The Master's Gift; is this ancient Qigong itself.

Qigong's Biggest Secret

Throughout this book we explain why Qigong, Floating Monk in particular, is so beneficial. We describe how Qigong improves circulation, enhances metabolism, and oxygenates the body. We also describe how the gentle, flowing movements of Floating Monk Qigong warm and strengthen the joints, and tone the body.

Traditional Chinese medicine prescribes Qigong for the treatment of numerous maladies. Hospitals in China have been incorporating Qigong into treatment programs for many years. In addition to the testimonials of Qigong practitioners, research into Qigong, going on for decades, shows overwhelmingly positive results. Yet for all of the evidence related to the benefits of practicing Qigong, there is rarely a whisper about Qigong's biggest secret.

Qigong's biggest secret has long been known by advanced practitioners, Sifus, and Masters, but it is rarely discussed publicly. It is rooted in the understanding or belief that there are two types of chi. The first type of chi is referred to as natural chi or life force. It is believed that we are all born with a certain amount of life force, and that once this supply is used up, it is gone forever. The second type of chi is referred to as acquired chi and, as the name implies, this chi is acquired from an outside source.

The only known means by which a person can obtain additional life force (chi) is believed to be through Qigong. This is Qigong's biggest secret. In high-level Qigong circles, this belief is considered to be a truth, and evidence of this truth is found in the long lives and healthy physical condition of Qigong Masters, as well as in the healing powers of certain Qigong practices.

Generally speaking, Qigong Masters and Sifus are not interested in challenging the principles they hold to be truths. Truths are self-evident; they are supported by the principles, practices, and simple logic of the Qigong programs. Truths are also closely held beliefs. Sifus and Masters are not interested in public scrutiny or clinical scientific examinations intent on debunking their beliefs, which is one of the reasons why Qigong's biggest secret is rarely, if ever, discussed.

The idea that Qigong can help a practitioner obtain additional life force is what makes it unique. We believe in the benefits of a variety of physical activities, from gardening to running, biking, yoga, walking, or cardiovascular and strengthening programs. Qigong is one of many options for improving health and prolonging life, but to our knowledge, it is the only program designed to enhance and increase our life force, our chi.

Ting Sing Qigong

Ting Sing Qigong is the name of the Qigong related to this specific pai (*Kwong Sai Jook Lum Gee Tong Long Pai*). Since this Qigong was never shown beyond the temple walls, the name Ting Sing is not allowed for a program being publicly shared. The world beyond the temple walls, especially the cities and towns, are sometimes referred to within the temples as the world of the red dust. Prior to the Master allowing this Qigong to be shared, Ting Sing has never been taught publicly in the world of the red dust.

The name Ting Sing remains inside the temple. For this reason, the name Floating Monk was adopted and is the name we use for this Qigong when showing and teaching it to the public. As was mentioned, in Chinese mythology the floating monks were known as the messengers of important information, and we felt this name was fitting because we were bringing this valuable information to the public for the very first time.

A Hundred Roads to Rome

We use the word Rome as a metaphor for a goal, a destination, or a place a person is seeking to reach physically, philosophically, or even spiritually. When teaching Qigong, we explain that there are a hundred roads to Rome. Rome (the destination) may represent peace of mind, a sense of calm, or a feeling of spiritual connection. It can also be a feeling of connection to our intuitive wisdom or our personal divine, which awaits us all; inside the quiet.

Not everyone prefers to travel the same road. Some people will prefer Floating Monk Qigong programs while others prefer yoga, dance, or various meditative practices. Some people find solace in running, biking, or fast, physically demanding fitness programs. While these programs provide a great many benefits, few programs work directly with the flow of our own internal life force (or chi) in addition to the internal and external benefits of Qigong.

You do not need to choose to practice Qigong over practicing some other program; perhaps one of the best approaches is to combine Qigong with activities you already do, especially as Qigong practice can be done in small increments of a few minutes, or as a complete exercise in fifteen to twenty minutes. Qigong works wonderfully with other more physically demanding activities.

Choosing the Road That's Right for You

The very next section will describe how the Floating Monk Qigong programs can help you to live a fuller, healthier, happier, and more energetic life. We sincerely hope that you find our programs of value and that you make a little time to enjoy them daily. If you choose another road or another program for your current path, we hope that you will enjoy it and find it fulfilling. We welcome your return if the future finds you once again upon this path.

"If I had to limit my advice on healthier living to just one tip, it would be—

To learn to breathe correctly"

Dr. Andrew Weil

Our Programs

Our system contains three specific Qigong platforms, they are: Sitting Qigong, Standing Qigong, and Stretching Qigong. The information within these programs is divided into the following levels:

Sitting Qigong   Levels I and II
Stretching Qigong   Levels I and II
Standing Qigong   Levels I, II, III, IV, V (level V is the Sifu level)

How You Benefit

Sitting Qigong

To the casual observer unfamiliar with Qigong, it would appear that a person doing Sitting Qigong is sitting still doing very little. The first part is true, they are sitting fairly still, although there is some movement, but the thought that they are doing very little would be completely incorrect.

Bruce Lee referred to meditation and Qigong type programs as active inactivity; from the outside it appears that very little is happening, while inside a great deal is happening. This effectively describes Floating Monk Sitting Qigong. The Sitting Qigong program is wonderful for people of any age. It is also an excellent program for businesses and organizations as it can be done in work attire.

Sitting Qigong is also very popular with those who have injured joints, muscles, or other health issues which make it uncomfortable to do the Standing Qigong. Medical and rehabilitation facilities, wellness centers, and senior activity centers also tend to favor the Sitting Qigong Program.

A Truly Unique Program

No other program uses the same sitting posture, hand and arm positions, and breathing techniques as Floating Monk Qigong. The information we provide about the flow of the breath, the movement of the chi through the body, the change in hand positions, and the transition from yin to yang and back to yin provides a clear, practical, and easy to follow series of movements, allowing even a first-time practitioner to enjoy and benefit from our programs.

In the first class alone, many students said they learned more than they had at the completion of other programs. After we guide beginning students into the proper body posture, we explain what the posture is designed to do, and how. We inform students about what they may experience and then we begin the practice of Sitting Qigong.

Standing Qigong

The Standing Qigong program is the central program of both Floating Monk and the original Ting Sing Qigong System. The Floating Monk Standing Qigong program has five levels; each level is needed due to the vast amount of information and technique in the complete program. The longer you train in Floating Monk, the more you come to understand and appreciate the depth of the knowledge, as well as the logic and practicality, behind each and every movement.

One of the most appreciated aspects of Floating Monk Qigong is that it builds upon the information and techniques of the previous levels.

This varies significantly from other Qigong programs which teach a new series of motions with every level.

In the beginning program, we teach practitioners how chi moves through the body in a circle. The Level I program introduces the idea of circular breathing, as well as the up and down movements, and explains how the movement coordinates with the breath to create a powerful sense of flowing energy throughout the body.

Level II Standing Qigong introduces what we call the Six Sections of the Circle. Practitioners then learn how to move various groups of muscles in coordination with the breath. This smooth, relaxed, synchronized movement creates an even more powerful Qigong experience.

Levels III, IV, and V

The most unique and powerful movements of the Floating Monk Qigong program are found in these levels. Level III and above are for individuals who want to experience Qigong in a way that they may not have previously imagined. We reserve the right to teach these levels to those who are serious about Qigong, especially those interested in teaching and helping us to bring the benefits of Floating Monk Qigong to more people.

How Much Qigong is Enough?

The first two levels of Floating Monk Qigong are the foundation for the higher levels. Understanding and effectively practicing the first two levels provides a vast amount of benefit to the practitioner, so the higher levels are not a necessity. If someone is truly determined to learn the higher levels, or they are committed to learning and teaching the first two levels of the program in partnership with Floating Monk, it is best to practice Levels I and II for some months before proceeding to the higher levels.

Grand Master Yee was very fond of telling students regarding the first two levels,

"If you learn this Qigong, and you practice regularly, you have enough Qigong for the rest of your life."

Stretching Qigong

The Sitting Qigong and the Standing Qigong are a direct reflection of the Ting Sing Qigong from which it originates. The Stretching Qigong encapsulates principles of the Ting Sing, but also information gleaned from Shaolin Kung Fu training and other related programs over more than thirty years.

One of the primary goals of the Stretching Qigong program is to teach the practitioner how to use the breath to have a conversation with the body. The timing of the inhale and the exhale are coordinated to specific movements.

Many long-time practitioners of other stretching and breathing programs have told us how much they appreciate the logic and organized flow of movements within this program.

The Series of Movements

The Stretching Qigong program warms and "oils" every joint in the body. The program begins with a twisting technique popular in Taoist internal cleansing programs. Once the body is warm, the Big Circles are next, followed by a stretch called Greet the Day. The next series stretches warms the large muscle groups in the front and back of the body, followed by long, relaxed side body stretches.

Once the series of stretches is complete, a series called The World of Circles follows, then the Windmill, side Windmills, and chest and back stretches with a few twists near the finish. The final movements of the Stretching Qigong are front and back leg stretches, followed by a few additional twists to complete the program and prepare you to meet the day.

Health from the Inside Out

Perhaps the best way to understand health from the inside out is to consider what it means to be healthy. Good health and overall vitality is predicated on all of the organs of the body working well independently, and in unison with one another. Have you ever seen an ad for a fitness program which talked about the health of your organs? The fact that you probably haven't underlies how health and wellness is perceived in Western culture.

In the West

In the West, many exercise advertisements show people in their early twenties to their early thirties wearing spandex and looking ripped as they jump, pump, bend, and sweat. There is nothing wrong with being physically fit, looking good, and feeling good about it. That's not the point. Congratulations to those who do such programs and enjoy them. The point is that Western exercise is often focused externally while the focus of Eastern wellness and fitness programs is from the inside out.

In the West, appearance is supreme. Fitness is frequently measured in terms of appearance; looking and acting young is favored over age, experience, and wisdom. Traditional Chinese medicine states that energy must be balanced and in a state of flow for an organism (or individual) to function properly and to flourish.

In the East

From an Eastern perspective, health is viewed much more from the inside out. In the East, evidence of good health is measured by clear skin and eyes, energy, vitality, and even by obtaining old age. Those who live well, exercise (which often includes Qigong), and achieve a healthy appearance and old age are revered, and their advice is sought by those who respect their age and wisdom.

It is neither fair nor wise to make bold claims, to say that one way is good and the other is bad. In the measurement of wellness, as in life, the truth is often somewhere in between. We understand and appreciate the benefits of Qigong and believe that a person of any age will feel better, healthier, and have more energy by practicing Qigong, but we also recognize that everyone must find their own way.

Ponce de Leon and the Search for the Fountain of Youth

When the Spanish explorer Ponce de Leon embarked on his famous voyages in search of the fountain of youth, he went looking externally, whereas he may have had better fortune by looking within. He may also have benefited from interviewing those who possessed the gift of health and old age, and considered both what they were doing internally, such as their diet, rather than focusing completely on a spring which contained the secret of eternal youth.

CHAPTER 10

Turning the Light to the Heart

MANY YEARS AGO, I was asked to come to Augusta to teach a workshop for a group of therapists. The sponsor was a physical therapist who owned and operated two clinics and had been on the faculty of the Medical College of Georgia, a prestigious school located in Augusta. The group consisted of doctors and accomplished practitioners in the mental health and physical therapy fields, among others.

As I walked into the room and sat down facing the group, there was an air of anticipation. I looked out at the group and one of the first things I told them was this:

"If you practice this Qigong program, you should prepare yourself because one of the effects of this practice is that it turns the light to your heart."

What I was trying to prepare them for was that the program they were about to learn would begin with what we call "turning off the noise." When you turn down or turn off the noise of life and chatter in your mind, you slowly enter into the quiet. You then naturally begin to ask yourself what is really important. This noise-free environment shifts the light (the attention) away from the chatter of your mind and toward those things which your heart truly desires and believes in.

Once this idea began to sink in amongst the crowd, I continued: "If you like the work you are doing, then you will love this Qigong because your inner-self is about to steer the light in that direction. If, however, you do not like what you are doing, if you are questioning your passion, or perhaps are unsure where your passion truly lies, you will be made aware of it as a result of this training. It is amazing what your heart will reveal to you when you turn your attention away from the daily chatter of your mind and toward your heart, meaning toward what you really love, enjoy, or want to do with your life.

If we were to replace the word "heart" with the word "soul" or "spirit," what we are saying here would take on a much deeper meaning. As you read and re-read this section about turning the light to your heart, consider the idea of soul or spirit and you may gain additional insight. We are using the term "light to your heart" because this is the way it is taught, however, as many of us know, Eastern philosophies often present ideas using terms and symbols which are easily understood or easy to relate to, but the idea, like an onion, may have many layers.

This same effect holds true for relationships. One of the things practitioners find when they begin our programs is a conscious awareness of what they value. This frequently evolves into an awareness of what they most value in their relationships; at work, with their spouse, and elsewhere in their lives.

What practitioners' desire most in a spouse or life partner is someone whose spiritual views, passions, and values are close to their own.

When we think about it, we often find ourselves saying: Of course, it's so simple, why did I not see that before? One reason, though there are many, that we may never have consciously considered this before is because we were trying so hard to be happy. Suddenly we see it and it all seems perfectly reasonable and clear. We are spiritual beings living in physical bodies. Naturally, we want to be happy, to meet and even exceed the necessities of physical existence (through our homes, jobs, cars, clothes, and other material items) but as spirits we know there is more to our current existence.

Qigong, while being an incredibly beneficial physical practice, is also one of many roads to greater spiritual awareness.

Shakespeare and Shaolin

"All the world is a stage, and all the men and women merely players."

(William Shakespeare, *As You like It*, Act 1, scene 1)

When we watch a play, we see what is occurring on the stage in front of the curtain, but if they were to pull back the curtain, we would see that there is a lot more going on than what we originally observed. Our programs are much like a stage play in this way; the practice is like the scene upon the stage, but the result, the experience, and the journey is similar to what occurs behind the curtain.

In our programs we use the term "conversation" quite frequently. In the Stretching Qigong program we talk about your breath having a conversation with your body. In Standing and Sitting Qigong, we talk about the conversation between your breath, your muscles, and your mind. On the first day of the first program, we talk about finding your place on the earth, and as the programs advance, we talk about the conversation between earth and heaven. The word heaven could be switched with the word cosmos, the conversation would still be the same.

Chi: Our Life Force

The energy that flows through the postures of the Qigong begins within our bodies, it is the energy of chi; our life force. Soon after learning how to circulate your own energy, we discuss drawing in and releasing the energy that surrounds you through the air we breathe. In time, we discuss the energy of earth and heaven, and how your body is a focal point and a conduit between the two.

Recognizing, nourishing, and participating in this flow of energy is what we call "the conversation." As the conversation becomes more active, through attentive practice, the energy expands. When this occurs, the energy goes outward and upward. Over time, your sense of awareness, intuition, and connection becomes stronger.

The Path toward Love

At Floating Monk, we neither teach nor profess any specific philosophical or religious belief, in part, because the very process of practicing these programs will lead you to your own insights. It has been our experience that whatever spiritual faith you hold within you, whatever source you consider your divine will become clearer and stronger as a result of entering into a conversation with the energy within, around, and beyond you.

We believe that every faith, life view, and philosophy will eventually meet on one central path, and that is the path towards love.

CHAPTER 11

From Oral History to Written Text, Training Manuals, and DVDs

Traditions

TRADITIONS, ONCE ESTABLISHED, remain as they are until someone changes them. In the world of Qigong, and much of martial arts, traditions are in many cases, hundreds, and in some cases, thousands of years old. One of the oldest traditions in the Qigong and Kung Fu world relates to passing on the secrets of a system from generation to generation, from one Master to the next.

In most cases, written information of some kind passes from one Master to the next, but in many cases, the Masters are the only ones who will ever see this information. Only recently have programs begun to produce written information. Even in recent times, programs will advertise publicly and provide brochures (with a brief bio of the Master/Instructor) when you visit the school, but that would often be the last time you would see anything about the system in print.

Most of the instruction in traditional schools is oral, from the history of the system, to the programs offered, to the levels within the programs. The programs themselves, including every movement in every form, is passed from teacher to student orally. This was the tradition and it was never questioned. If you did talk about it privately with your classmates you never considered asking the Master why more of the information was not in written form.

An Entire System

Imagine for a Moment what it would be like to write out each and every movement of a form that took just a minute or two to perform. It may not sound too difficult, but as soon as you begin describing every hand, elbow, shoulder, waist, ankle, and knee motion for a single set of movements, you soon realize that the task is far bigger and much more laborious than you had initially imagined. It is almost an impossible task.

In addition to the motion itself, now consider explaining what the breath is doing, and what the muscles are doing, besides the movement. Now add the intent, where your mind is focused (or not focused) while you are performing each technique and suddenly you begin to understand the scope of such an undertaking.

This is one of the reasons that so little of the information on Qigong and Kung Fu programs is written down. If a program is generous enough to write out what it offers, and provides some information about the levels within the program, you should consider yourself fortunate.

Student Notebooks

Much of the specific information about various forms, and the nuances within the forms, can only be found in two places; the first place is in the Master's mind and the second place is within the pages of the student's notebooks. We were sometimes allowed to break away during our training to make notes about a new form or a particular technique. At other times, especially when the Master was talking, we knew better than to even ask. At those times we did our very best to listen closely, knowing we would make our notes later.

Teaching is Learning

It has often been said that the best way to learn something is to teach it. I firmly believe in this approach. No matter how well you think you know something, you will never be sure until the Moment you try to teach it. When you have to explain the order of a particular series of motions, and begin to take questions or provide explanations regarding why something is done, or not done, a particular way, you begin to appreciate what it means to truly know something well.

In teaching, you must revisit everything you have ever learned about the given subject. You go back and study your notes, and you mentally review what it was like when you were trying to learn a form or technique for the first time. You find that you have to think deeper; you think through what a form or a technique is trying to accomplish, and you realize that you have to know the entire system far more intimately than before.

You begin to realize that you cannot merely *teach Qigong*, you have to *become Qigong*. That is where the journey truly begins. You probably won't realize it at the time, but once you start down that path, you will never return as the same person as when the journey first began.

Ting Sing Qigong had an Oral History

When the Master gave permission to take this Qigong out into the world, allowing it to be shown to the public for the first time, it existed entirely in oral history. There was not a single word related to any technique or form written down anywhere, except in student notebooks. In addition, the system had been taught layer by layer over a period of many years, and during this time additional techniques were added to specific sections, techniques that were alternates for other techniques.

This Qigong had always been taught as part of a Kung Fu system, and then only to the serious long-term practitioners or students of the Master. The Qigong was totally separate and unique from Kung Fu, but we were used to learning this way; getting little pieces of information over a period of many years. The way that we had learned Qigong was unique; it was not a process that could be used in teaching to the public. An entirely new approach had to be developed.

Initial Efforts

I had already been teaching Qigong to Kung Fu students I was training privately and in groups for many years. We were always allowed to teach the Qigong as a part of Kung Fu, but, with the Master's recent permission, I would now be teaching Qigong as a separate program. Martial arts instructors I had known for many years, as well as friends and relatives of my private students, became my first students.

I monitored the results as I taught, watching for progress week by week. I soon realized what I considered to be an error in the way that I was teaching.

I was teaching the program in much the same way that I had learned and was practicing it, and that was the error. When I began to learn Qigong, I had already been training Kung Fu for many years, so I understood the terminology, and the movements came naturally to me.

These new students did not have such references, so the amount of information I was giving them was both too extensive and too advanced. I realized that I would have to dissect the entire program and rebuild it. Once the fundamentals were in place, the students would have a foundation and I would be able to slowly add new information.

Beginning at Square One

I began by categorizing the programs into Sitting, Standing, and Stretching Qigong. The process of breaking down and recording all of the techniques took a very long time, but it was absolutely essential to do it this way. I had to determine where the line was between one level and the next.

Initially, I structured the information into three levels, but the amount of information on each level was still too great, and the process of learning even the first level took far too long. I had to go back and dissect the information again, to make each level less arduous and more enjoyable to learn. Once this task was complete, years after the first efforts had begun, the process was complete; there were now five levels, and that is the way the program remains structured to this day.

CHAPTER 12

Our Partners and Supporters

AS A STUDENT, when you consider beginning any new program, it is comforting to know that others have walked the path before you, especially when they are willing to discuss their experience with you. This feeling is similar to starting a new job and knowing that you have one or more friends working at the company, that you can have lunch with them sometimes, and that you may even work together in the same department. Regardless of the circumstances, the main point is that you don't feel so alone.

For this reason, we felt that you would like to know what some of today's well known doctors and wellness personalities have to say about programs such as ours. We also thought that you would like to hear from others who have personally experienced our program, including doctors, chiropractors, a physical therapist from the faculty of a noted medical college, registered nurses, massage therapists, a noted acupuncturist and wellness coach, as well as an attorney, pilot, world-renowned chef, and the director of a corporate wellness program.

> "I believe these focused breathing techniques are beneficial in reducing work-related stress. Participants sited increased energy and a greater feeling of relaxation."
>
> Lori K. Cook, regional program coordinator, Northrop Grumman
> IT Heat Waves Wellness Program

In a business environment, whether a company has five employees or five thousand, wellness and prevention are the only two areas where employers have any possible input. Medical care costs continue to rise and no business has the ability to change this. It is fiducially responsible and financially practical for companies to implement a wellness approach to their overall health-care offering.

Not only is this a financially logical approach for businesses, as the wellness of its employees have a direct impact on every business' bottom line, it is also a responsible way for a business to show its employees that they truly care. Businesses understand that in order to remain viable, dollars in must exceed dollars out, and wellness and preventative care programs can positively and directly address this issue.

"I have found that just fifteen minutes of deep breathing would give one all the energy they need for the day.

The better you feel, the more you use your talent to produce outstanding results."

Tony Robbins

"I work long hours focusing on detailed information. Doing just a few minutes of Qigong as I sit at my desk eases the stress, helps me to focus, and gives me the energy to continue."

Mike Crawford, attorney at law, Atlanta, Georgia

"The energy and focus I experience from doing Qigong exceeded my expectations.

I can't imagine beginning my day without it."

Guenter Seeger, Michelin five-star chef and consultant

From Medical and Wellness Professionals Who Have Personally Experienced our Programs

"I have been a physical therapist for over twenty-five years, including time on the faculty at the Medical College of Georgia. When I saw Floating Monk Qigong and listened to Sifu Jeff explain how and why it works, I knew immediately that I had found something of real value. I do the program myself and am integrating it into my practice. I recommend this program to other physical therapy practitioners, medical doctors, and anyone in the business of health and healing."

Jurgen D. Cowling, owner/president: Healing Hands Therapy Centers, Augusta, Georgia

"As a doctor of Western medicine and a practitioner of Qigong, I find that medical definitions lack the vocabulary to encompass the workings and benefits of Qigong. I have felt an increased sense of health and vitality from practicing Qigong. I think that in order to grasp what Qigong is about, it requires participation. It is an excellent endeavor for anyone, young or old, who is seeking a well-rounded way to improve and maintain their health."

Chris Carlson, M.D., surgeon, Trinity Medical Group, Augusta, Georgia

Some Qigong practitioners have experienced such benefits as: Reduced stress, greater stamina, enhanced mental clarity, greater awareness, calmness, and an overall sense of well-being.

*Web*MD

Our experience with the Floating Monk Qigong program was extremely positive. The program was simple and the exercises were modified a little so that everyone in our group could participate. Though the breathing exercises were comfortable and easy to do, they were intense enough that it felt like we had run miles when we were through; your heart rate felt great, you could breathe normally, your brain had enough oxygen flow, your entire body felt the workout, and you were energized after every session. We all loved it.

Sifu Jeff, a wholesome, kind, and gentle giant, brought this resource to us in an act of kindness and goodwill. He and Sifu Jim were awesome professionals who knew their craft. The candidates in our program learned that they could do their breathing exercises while driving, cooking, at work, or relaxing at home and every breath taken was an awesome feeling. Weight control with breathing exercises did not feel intimidating, even to the heaviest candidates; they could do the exercises and gained enormous benefits from the sessions.

I highly recommend the Floating Monk Qigong program, but especially Sifu Jeff. He is an amazing man, an amazing professional, and a highly skilled individual who is sincere about helping folks lead healthy lifestyles. Sifu Jim was also an incredible teacher, his unique coaching program helped our entire group to reach insights they can use in both their careers and their personal lives.

Cindy Williams, PhD, founder, Women Are Dreamers Too

> "Qigong can help us stretch, stay loose, and balance both mind and body.
>
> It allows us to cope with the day-to-day struggles of being human."
>
> Dr. Oz

Additional Information

For more information about our partners and supporters, as well as a list of the groups, organizations, and businesses that have participated in our programs, please visit: floatingmonk.com.

CHAPTER 13

Vision and Outreach

From the Ancient World to the Modern Day

F ROM A PUBLIC perspective, Qigong is still relatively unknown. Our hope in writing this book is to provide a simple, clear, and understandable explanation of Qigong, where it came from, and how it can benefit people.

The vision for Floating Monk is to provide Qigong information, education, and training to the general public, businesses, and organizations. Qigong is our passion. We are convinced that Qigong can bring significant physical, mental, and spiritual benefits to those who practice regularly.

Ancient Traditions

The ancient traditions are an intriguing aspect of Qigong. In our workshops, students have always shown great enthusiasm for learning about and discussing the ancient traditions. The Unspoken Codes and Who's Your Sifu are two important aspects of the ancient traditions. The codes provide anyone interested in learning Qigong with a way to qualify potential programs and instructors, and help potential students understand what qualities and certifications a potential teacher should possess.

Discussing the Unspoken Codes and other Taoist and Buddhist principles helps the reader to understand the values and principles of the ancient ways. As we discuss learning, understanding, and applying ancient wisdom, we believe it is important to know where the wisdom came from and why it is revered.

Floating Monk's Outreach Program

Our outreach program provides information, education, and training related to Qigong, as well as information, services, and support in the chi-based coaching programs we offer. Finally, we hope to serve as an information source for Qigong and other programs related to health and wellness.

Wellness

Wellness is the central focus of all Floating Monk programs; wellness of spirit, of mind, and body. Our Sitting, Standing, and Stretching Qigong programs all address these important areas, and assist practitioners toward achieving their vision and their goals.

Our Website

Our website provides detailed information about our Qigong and coaching programs and training, as well as informational DVDs, downloads and other materials. We also provide detailed written material to assist in understanding each of our programs.

Classes and Workshops

Information about our classes and workshops is available on our website. Classes and workshops are ongoing in Minneapolis, Minnesota and Atlanta, Georgia, and plans for other U.S. cities, Canada, and Europe. It is our desire to make our programs available to everyone, regardless of economics. To achieve this, many of our Minneapolis classes, and some of our workshops are offered by donation, with no set cost.

Other Programs

Our website provides links to other programs we support, such as those offered at the Ahimki Center in Roswell, Georgia, by Sifu Dr. Mark Armstrong. Find out more about Dr. Mark's programs at www.Ahimki.net

To Complement or Enhance the Qigong Experience

We also provide links to other sites which can benefit practitioners of our programs and Qigong practitioners in general. In addition, we make items available on our website which we believe can enhance or complement health, wellness, and the overall Qigong experience.

Sifu Jeff Larson

Sifu Jeff manages all the training programs offered by Floating Monk. This includes classes and workshops for those just beginning Qigong, as well as the instructor training workshops. Sifu Jeff frequently travels to assist individuals and organizations seeking the benefit of the Floating Monk programs.

Sifu Jim Beasley

Sifu Jim manages all the coaching programs. Sifu Jim offers coaching for individuals and groups. Sifu Jim has designed a special, certified coaching program based on the principles and practices of Qigong. This turn-key program is available to those who wish to add coaching to their current wellness services.

Sifu Jim also has similar, certified programs for practicing coaches who wish to add a unique, inwardly focused coaching aspect to their current practice. For more information and a complete list of programs please visit our website.

For More Information

We welcome you to visit our website www.floatingmonk.com for detailed information about our various programs and services. We look forward to being of service.

Author Biographies

JIM BEASLEY is a professional coach and business and real estate consultant. Over the last fifteen years he has worked with local, regional, and national organizations, including NASA, IBM, the FBI, and EEOC. His work has been featured in *Consulting Today, the International Coaching Federation Journal, the Atlanta Journal Constitution*, and *The Coaching Revolution* by John King and David Logan.

Jim has more than twenty-five years of experience in the martial arts. He is an internationally certified black belt chief instructor and Qigong black sash sifu.

He has studied and trained in alternative healing modalities for more than fifteen years under two well-known healers: Dorothy Spitler and Dr. Walter Weston. He is trained in energetic healing, spiritual healing, emotional relief therapy, distance healing, and laying on of hands. Jim was featured in Dr. Weston's book *Emotional Relief Therapy: Letting Go of Life's Painful Emotions.*

Some of Sifu Jim's achievements include:

AA, JD, Graduate Fellow the Institute for Court Management, Graduate Coach University.

From Jim's Clients

"Over the last eighteen months, I was able to experience what masterful coaching feels like to a client, and have drawn from that experience to create the same atmosphere for my clients."
Senior coach, fortune 50 company

"You have had a big impact on me and the company. Our team atmosphere has been restored."
Commercial electrical contracting firm, Atlanta, Georgia

"Our morale is up and our stress is down."
Manager, EEOC, United States Government

"The information you presented and the clarity with which you did so, gave me the motivation and resources I needed to begin my venture."
College administrator, Atlanta, Georgia

"The only time I focus on my life is when we meet. I really get clear on the direction I want to take and the action necessary to get there."
Business owner, Denver, Colorado

"I always wanted to experience a miracle of healing—today I did."
Leadership Executive, San Francisco, California

Sifu Jeff Larson is a recognized and respected instructor of Qigong and Kung Fu. He has been teaching classes, workshops, group programs, and individual (private) students for over a quarter of a century. His private students include many recognized and respected individuals in the world of business, medicine, and the arts. He believes that every student matters and that the impact of the Qigong they learn resonates within their personal lives, as well as in the communities where they live and work.

Sifu Jeff has demonstrated and taught Qigong at numerous venues, and has won gold and silver medals in Qigong and martial arts at the regional, national, and international level. He has also trained students and instructors who have become gold and silver medal winners. Teaching is his passion, and one of his goals is to teach students and teachers across North America, Europe, and beyond. Sifu Jeff is a certified black sash in Qigong and Kung Fu. He is an Enter the Gate Disciple of his respected Sifu: Grand Master Henry Poo Yee.

Sifu Jeff firmly believes in helping others to enhance their awareness and improve their lives. We all have something to offer each other and our communities, and the sharing of knowledge and services connects and helps to advance us all. In addition to his role as a Qigong teacher, energy coach, and healer, Sifu Jeff has a BA in Finance and an MBA, and has been working as an independent financial advisor for more than 15 years.

As an organization, Floating Monk's focus is service to others, and helping people to achieve and experience the fullness of their potential. Qigong is the foundation of our organization and it is an incredible tool, but we believe that affiliation with other programs and organizations can be helpful in our efforts to serve the communities in which we live.

From Jeff's Clients

I had never heard of Qigong and had no idea what it was, until Sifu Jeff introduced it to me during one of my private Kung Fu classes with him. I am a skeptic, I don't believe a lot of the programs out there which talk about energy, but this Qigong was different. I could actually feel the energy in my body, and when Sifu Jeff had me pause as he corrected my form, I honestly felt the difference it made.

Keith Clegg. Pilot Atlanta, GA

Sifu Jeff talks about how the Qigong cleanses your body, how it makes you feel clean, I know it sounds strange, but in addition to the energy it gives me, I actually felt clean from doing the Qigong. It's an amazing feeling.

Nico Ward. Actress Atlanta, GA

Qigong leads one to universal truth. Qigong, like breath, is not something you own; you incorporate it into your daily life with greater awareness. The more you are aware of maximizing your breathing, the healthier you become.

Sifu Pascal Sellem (CAI) Celebrity Hair Salon Atlanta GA

CHAPTER 14

Conclusion

History

ONE OF THE central themes throughout this book has been history. We have talked about the history of Qigong in general, the history of this system of Qigong, and of the Master of the system, Grand Master Henry Poo Yee, who has allowed us to share this information with you. We have discussed the idea of people being born in their time, or at a point in history when what they contribute has a potentially significant influence upon us as individuals, a society, and as a human family.

History is the great educator. Poets, philosophers, painters, and musicians are all fond of history. Through their gifts of reflection in essays, poetry, painting, and song, we feel the pulse and power of our own lives and the feeling of community with the generations to which we belong.

It is difficult or even impossible to measure the influence of such individuals as Mahatma Gandhi, Martin Luther King Jr., John F. Kennedy, Wolfgang Amadeus Mozart, Vincent Van Gogh, Robert Frost, Albert Einstein, and an endless list of others, until their lives are over and their influence is fully recognized.

Ancient Wisdom and Modern Life

The Qigong which the Grand Master has allowed us to show to the public could not have been timelier. The simplicity of the motions, and the easy, relaxed breathing techniques, allows the very young to the very old to learn and benefit from these programs. As the founders of the Floating Monk series of programs, we feel honored and extremely fortunate to be able to offer the world so great a gift at a time when its benefits are so needed.

By giving his permission, Grand Master Yee demonstrates what it means to be of service to others, and to reflect the light, wisdom and knowledge of those who came before us. We believe that his lifelong efforts to teach, preserve, and advance his art and the CKFA system will surely place his footprints upon the sands of time.

With humility, respect and dedication to my Sifu.

Grand Master Henry Poo Yee

"I have a great teacher."

Sifu Jeff Larson

We would like to finish this book with these words:

Thank you for your interest in our book. We hope that the information we provided, and the stories we shared have been interesting, informative, and entertaining, but most of all, we hope that you enjoyed what we've provided and feel that this information has brought value to your life. Perhaps all of us, in consideration of the many gifts we have to offer one another, were born into our time.

Floating Monk

Website: FloatingMonk.com
Email: FloatingMonk@live.com
Phone: (404) 323-6856

Authors are credited directly beneath all quotes used in this book

www.ingramcontent.com/pod-product-compliance
Lightning Source LLC
Chambersburg PA
CBHW020339290526
45785CB00005B/2088